THE MEDICINE-FREE,
ILLNESS-FREE SERIES

ANIMAL ORGAN
THERAPY

The Most Nutrient-Rich Superfoods for Organ
Health, Hormonal Balance, and Energy

Forest Yin, DAOM, L.Ac.

Ashi Healing Publishing

First Edition: May 2025

Published by Ashi Healing

www.AshiHealing.com

Paperback ISBN: 978-1-967735-06-8

eBook ISBN: 978-1-967735-07-5

Printed in the United States of America

Medical Disclaimer:

This book is for informational purposes only and is not intended as medical advice. The author and publisher assume no responsibility for how the information is used. Readers should consult a healthcare professional before making any health-related decisions.

Foreword

Nature is the origin of life, the origin of healing, and remains a guiding force in human well-being. Long before modern science developed medicine in laboratories, nature provided everything the human body needed to survive, and to sustain life. The food we eat, the herbs we gather, the minerals beneath our feet, and the sun above us are all part of an intelligent and interconnected system that has long nourished and supported the human body.

This truth has been known across cultures for thousands of years, and it is echoed in sacred texts. In the Book of Genesis, the Garden of Eden was described as a paradise where "every tree that is pleasant to the sight and good for food" was made available to humankind (Genesis 2:9). Some scholars believe this refers not only to nourishment, but also to the ability to contribute to human well-being. It becomes even more clear in Ezekiel 47:12: "The fruit thereof shall be for meat, and the leaf thereof for medicine."

Somewhere along the way, modern culture drifted from this wisdom. Many now believe that healing must come through synthetic drugs, surgeries, or man-made interventions, forgetting that the foundation of human health has always been rooted in nature. But what if well-being isn't only about medical breakthroughs, but also about reconnecting with what has always been available to us?

What if the body doesn't need to be forced to function differently, but simply supported, nourished, balanced, and reminded of what it already knows? What if illness is not the enemy, but a signal that we've fallen out of balance, and out of sync with nature?

This is not to dismiss the value of conventional medicine. We are deeply grateful for its life-saving capabilities in emergencies and acute care. But when it comes to supporting long-term vitality and encouraging balance, it may be time to return to the source.

In addition to thousands of years of lived wisdom, modern science is now exploring the potential of many natural approaches. What was once viewed as "alternative" is now increasingly recognized as part of a broader wellness conversation.

This book, and the entire *Medicine-Free, Illness-Free Series*, is rooted in this truth:

Nature not only gave us life. Many believe it holds the power to support our well-being. And many of these natural approaches are now being studied and better understood through science.

Healing is not something we must force or fear. It is something we can encourage, by gently supporting the body, naturally.

Dr. Forest Yin, DAOM, L.Ac.

Author, *The Medicine-Free, Illness-Free Series*

Founder, Ashi Healing and Acupuncture Inc.

Important Disclaimer

The supplements, therapies, and natural approaches discussed in *The Medicine-Free, Illness-Free Series* are intended to support general wellness and the body's natural balance. They are not intended to diagnose, treat, cure, or prevent any disease and have not been evaluated by the U.S. Food and Drug Administration (FDA).

These books are provided for educational purposes only and are not a substitute for professional medical advice, diagnosis, or treatment. Always consult your physician or a licensed healthcare provider before starting any new supplement, therapy, or wellness routine, especially if you are pregnant, nursing, have a medical condition, or are taking medications.

The content in this series is informed by two sources: summaries of available scientific research, presented as "Science-Informed Solution Benefits", and aggregated user feedback, presented as "Customer-Reported Solution Benefits". These are intended to inform and inspire, but they reflect general patterns, not guarantees. Individual results will vary.

The phrase *"Medicine-Free, Illness-Free"* reflects a natural wellness philosophy and is not a medical claim or promise of outcome.

By reading this book, you agree to take full responsibility for your personal health choices and to seek guidance from qualified health professionals when needed.

Contents

Preface

Do you feel like you've tried everything—medications, conventional treatments, even supplements—yet still struggle with fatigue, discomfort, brain fog, or other daily wellness concerns?

If so, you're not alone.

Many people today are turning to nature-based solutions, not as replacements for essential medical care, but as gentle, sustainable ways to support their overall well-being.

The rise in chronic health challenges reflects this shift. According to the CDC, over 60% of U.S. adults live with at least one chronic health condition, and more than 40% manage two or more. More than 40% of school-aged children in the United States are reported to have at least one ongoing wellness concern, rising sharply in recent years.

At the same time, modern habits, nutrient-depleted diets, environmental stressors, and sedentary routines, have created a disconnect between how we live and what the body truly needs to stay resilient. For many, conventional solutions haven't fully addressed these patterns, leaving people still searching for support that feels both effective and sustainable.

That's what *The Medicine-Free, Illness-Free Series* is here to explore.

This series introduces practical, natural options that may help support energy, digestion, sleep, focus, mood, and more, without requiring major lifestyle changes or complicated routines.

It doesn't reject conventional medicine. It expands your toolkit. While modern treatments often focus on managing symptoms in the short term, natural health practices are designed to work more gradually, supporting the body's natural rhythms over time. Many people are rediscovering how ancient practices and modern science can work together, not in opposition, to create a more balanced, resilient life.

The Medicine-Free, Illness-Free Series is built on two foundational pillars:

Science-Informed Solution Benefits: exploring what modern research says about the potential benefits associated with each supplement or therapy

Customer-Reported Solution Benefits: drawn from thousands of real-world user feedback to highlight what people most often experience in practice, including common benefit themes, typical use case patterns, and key user insights.

By combining scientific research with traditional use and real-world user feedback, each volume empowers you to make informed decisions, grounded in both evidence and everyday reality.

Each book in the series focuses on one category of natural therapies. Whether you're exploring Herbal Therapy, Mushroom Therapy, Amino Acid support, Animal Organ Supplements, Grounding, the HOPED Protocol, or detoxification, the goal is the same: to offer trusted solutions that fit easily into your life, simply, naturally, and sustainably.

You don't need to overhaul your lifestyle or commit to an elaborate health plan. You can begin right where you are. Even one small step, a single herb, nutrient, or daily practice, can help you create a rhythm of care that supports your body more naturally over time.

While no approach guarantees results, many people have found these natural strategies helpful in supporting comfort, energy, focus, and overall vitality. This series was created to help you explore those tools with clarity and confidence, without pressure or complexity.

This volume focuses on Animal Organ Therapy, offering practical insight into some of the most nutrient-dense organ extracts used for modern wellness. You'll learn about each organ through both research and real-world perspectives, so you can decide what feels right for your journey.

Thank you for beginning this exploration.

Let's move forward, one natural step at a time.

The Medicine-Free, Illness-Free Series

The Medicine-Free, Illness-Free Series is your go-to resource for practical, research-informed natural strategies that are easy to apply. Each volume focuses on a single modality or system—herbs, mushrooms, organ supplements, amino acids, grounding, detox, and more—offering clear guidance to help you choose what works best for you.

Together, the 10 books provide a comprehensive yet flexible wellness framework that supports both daily health maintenance and targeted support. Here's a brief overview of what you'll find in each book:

The Medicine-Free, Illness-Free Series: Why Natural Health Is the Future

Explore why millions of people are turning to nature-aligned strategies to support their wellness. This foundational volume introduces the core science and philosophy behind natural approaches to health, and how they may support your sense of balance, vitality, and overall well-being.

The Medicine-Free, Illness-Free Series: Herbal Therapy

Learn how the world's most time-tested plants may support digestion, energy, relaxation, immune strength, and more. Discover practical ways to include them in your routine and how to choose herbs that match your personal needs and constitution.

The Medicine-Free, Illness-Free Series: Mushroom Therapy

Discover the unique compounds found in medicinal mushrooms that may support immunity, cognitive function, and stress resilience. This book explains how to use mushrooms such as Reishi, Lion's Mane, and Cordyceps in a daily supplement.

The Medicine-Free, Illness-Free Series: Animal Organ Therapy

Explore how nutrient-dense organ supplements, like liver, heart, and kidney, may provide highly bioavailable vitamins, minerals, and peptides. Learn how these traditional foods may support foundational wellness in areas like energy, endurance, and metabolic balance.

The Medicine-Free, Illness-Free Series: Amino Acid Therapy

Uncover the role of amino acids, the building blocks of life, in supporting mood, focus, muscle strength, and nervous system health. This volume shows how targeted amino acid support may help restore clarity, resilience, and emotional well-being.

The Medicine-Free, Illness-Free Series: HOPED Protocol

Learn the five foundational nutrient categories—High Fiber, Omega-3s & Antioxidants, Probiotics, Enzymes, and Vitamin D—and how to implement them as a core wellness strategy. HOPED is simple, actionable, and designed for everyday consistency.

The Medicine-Free, Illness-Free Series: Detoxification Therapy

Discover a gentle, nature-based approach to support your body's natural detoxification processes, promote balance, and encourage overall vitality using simple, practical techniques.

The Medicine-Free, Illness-Free Series: Grounding Therapy

Explore the science and practice of grounding (earthing), the natural process of reconnecting with the Earth's electrical field. Learn how this subtle practice may help support nervous system regulation, sleep quality, and emotional balance.

The Medicine-Free, Illness-Free Series: Diet, Lifestyle and Emotional Well-being

While drastic changes are not required, this volume introduces simple habits that promote long-term balance, covering food, movement, sleep, and emotional self-regulation in a way that aligns with the rest of your natural health plan.

The Medicine-Free, Illness-Free Series: Integrative Therapies for Everyday Health

This final volume brings together insights from the entire series, offering user-reported tools to help support everyday wellness goals, such as energy, digestion, sleep, immunity, and emotional resilience. It serves as a cross-reference for applying the therapies in complementary ways, helping you navigate your health journey with clarity and confidence.

Meet Dr. Forest Yin, DAOM, L.Ac.

Professionally known as Forest Yin, my official name is Jie Yin, while also known as 尹明杰 in the Chinese speaking communities.

For most of my professional life, I was known as a high-tech executive, problem-solver, and innovator in information security and technologies. In leadership roles at Oracle, Schwab, and Wells Fargo, I developed and managed advanced security solutions, ensuring stability, efficiency, and high performance in a fast-paced, high-stakes environment.

But after work, I was deeply immersed in another world, the science of natural health.

My journey into Traditional Chinese Medicine (TCM) began in college, when I first studied the *Huang Di Nei Jing (Yellow Emperor's Classic of Internal Medicine)* alongside my Physics degree. While excelling in my tech career, I continued to research, experiment, and apply natural healing principles, seeking ways to optimize health, energy, and resilience, not just for myself, but for those around me.

Recognizing the profound impact of natural medicine on long-term health and performance, I pursued formal training, becoming a Licensed Acupuncturist (L.Ac.) in 2018 and earning my Doctorate in Acupuncture and Oriental Medicine (DAOM) in 2019. Since then, I have supported individuals around the world in improving their vitality, resilience, and sense of well-being through natural methods. This led me to found Ashi Healing and Acupuncture Inc. and become a Professor and Doctoral Advisor at the University of East-West Medicine, where I mentor future practitioners in the art of TCM.

Applying Systems Thinking to Health & Healing

In high-tech, solving problems requires understanding systems, identifying vulnerabilities, and optimizing performance. I apply the same mindset to health. Instead of treating symptoms, I look at the root cause, like debugging a system. Instead of temporary fixes, I focus on long-term balance and resilience, like designing sustainable architecture. Instead of pharmaceutical dependency, I seek efficient, natural approaches that support function and balance gently, without the common side effects associated with conventional options, like optimizing system performance.

While many of my colleagues in the tech and finance industries thrived in their careers, I also saw the toll of chronic stress, burnout, autoimmune conditions, and lifestyle-related illnesses. Like many professionals, they pushed their limits, until their bodies pushed back. This is where natural approaches can make a difference.

A Philosophy Rooted in Balance & Natural Healing

At Ashi Healing, my approach complements conventional care by focusing on identifying underlying imbalances and supporting the body's natural self-regulation through Traditional Chinese Medicine and holistic strategies.

The name "Ashi (阿是)" comes from a fundamental concept in Chinese medicine, that moment of realization when healing feels real. In Chinese, "Ashi" means "Ahh, Yes!", the instant when your body recognizes exactly what it needs. This guiding philosophy shapes everything I do, from acupuncture to natural health solutions.

Through the precise use of Chinese Herbal Medicine and modern whole-food-based natural supplements like herbs and mushrooms, I have helped individuals support their energy and balance naturally, using simple, sustainable tools that complement or reduce the need for pharmaceutical interventions when appropriate.

My mission is simple: to help people pursue wellness and resilience, naturally and sustainably.

Integrating Ancient Wisdom with Modern Innovation

Chinese Herbal Medicine has been refined for thousands of years. But today, we can take it further, combining ancient wisdom with modern research and a strategic, data-driven approach to health optimization.

At Ashi Healing, I personalize each protocol based on the individual's needs, whether it's boosting energy, reducing stress, improving cognitive function, or addressing chronic health concerns. Many of the people I work with are busy professionals seeking practical, time-efficient strategies to support their health without disrupting their demanding schedules.

Looking for More Information and Support

To learn more about my personalized approach to Chinese Herbal Therapy and whole-food-based supplements, visit AshiHealing.com. You'll find additional resources and simple ways to take the next step in your healing journey, whenever you're ready.

And remember, this book is just one part of *The Medicine-Free, Illness-Free Series*. Each volume explores a different pillar of natural healing, from herbs and mushrooms to amino acids, detoxification, and grounding, offering you a complete path to support your balance and well-being through nature-based strategies.

A Science-Backed, Real-World Tested Method

In *The Medicine-Free, Illness-Free Series*, we introduce a unique, structured method for exploring natural supplements, one that blends scientific insight with real-world observations. Rather than relying solely on clinical studies or anecdotal reports, we combine both perspectives to give you a well-rounded, user-friendly understanding of each natural solution.

This balanced approach helps answer the most important questions: What does science suggest about this supplement's potential? What are people actually experiencing when they use it? Which health goals do people turn to it for most often?

Our method reflects a commitment to transparency, education, and practicality, so you can explore these natural options with clarity and confidence.

Our Four-Part Analysis Method

1. Science-Informed Solution Benefits

We begin by reviewing peer-reviewed studies, traditional usage patterns, and emerging scientific literature to understand the possible mechanisms and effects of each supplement. This provides a foundation of what is known, hypothesized, or being actively researched, offering a science-informed perspective to guide your exploration.

2. Customer-Reported Solution Benefits

13

We analyze large sets of customer reviews from publicly available platforms to understand how these supplements are being used in daily life. This includes what benefits people say they notice most often and how they describe their experiences.

Our focus is on patterns of what users commonly report, rather than isolated stories. This real-world layer helps connect the theory to practical, everyday outcomes.

3. Use Case Patterns & Feedback Insights

Within the customer-reported section, we highlight:

Use Case Patterns Observed – What kinds of goals or wellness concerns people most commonly use each supplement for.

Feedback Insights – How users describe the impact in their own words, including sentiment, language tone, and satisfaction cues.

Most Reported Benefits – A percentage-based summary showing which benefits are mentioned most often in reviews.

This structured summary lets you see what real people are using the supplement for, and how frequently those benefits are reported.

4. No Brand Promotion—Just Trusted Guidance

This series does not promote specific products or brands. Instead, we offer education and a decision-making framework. For those looking for high-quality sources, recommended supplement types and vetted options are available at AshiHealing.com.

Why This Method Matters

In today's crowded supplement market, it can be hard to separate hype from helpful information. That's why we created this approach, to empower you with insights drawn from scientific research, real-world usage patterns and satisfaction trends, and clear summaries that help you compare options and set expectations

You won't find exaggerated claims or one-size-fits-all solutions here. Instead, you'll find a practical, transparent method that reflects how real people are exploring natural wellness, with science as a guide and personal experience as a reference.

Whether you're considering herbs, mushrooms, amino acids, or other supplements, this method gives you a safe and structured way to learn how others are using these tools, and how they might fit into your own wellness journey.

A Personal Commitment from Dr. Forest Yin

Every approach, strategy, and supplement featured in *The Medicine-Free, Illness-Free Series* has been personally explored. Before sharing any recommendations with clients or readers, I take the time to experience it myself, observing how it affects energy, mood, sleep, digestion, and focus.

This hands-on approach allows me to understand each therapy not just through science, or just through other people's experiences. It adds a personal layer of insight to the research and user-reported feedback that shape this series.

My goal is simple: to help you find natural, sustainable solutions that feel doable, helpful, and aligned with how lasting wellness begins, by reconnecting with your body's own rhythms and innate intelligence.

The Power of
Animal Organ Therapy

For centuries, traditional cultures across the globe valued organ meats as some of the most nourishing and vital parts of the animal. Today, this ancient respect is experiencing a modern revival. Many people are rediscovering the nutritional richness of animal organs, not by preparing them in the kitchen, but through easy-to-use, shelf-stable supplements. This chapter introduces the philosophy, history, and growing popularity of grass-fed organ supplements, exploring why they have become a trusted option in today's wellness landscape.

A Return to Ancestral Wisdom

Throughout human history, animal organs were considered some of the most vital and nourishing parts of the animal. Across continents and cultures, from ancient Egypt and China to Indigenous communities in the Arctic and Africa, organ meats were not only consumed for survival but were revered for their symbolic and nutritional significance. These traditions were based on generations of observation and experience, often reflecting a deep intuitive understanding of which foods could sustain strength, vitality, and resilience.

In Traditional Chinese Medicine, animal organs were believed to support corresponding systems in the human body, a philosophy echoed in ancient Greek and Ayurvedic teachings. This "like supports like" concept guided the consumption of specific organs, such as liver for blood health or kidney for reproductive balance, as part of broader healing practices. Though rooted in traditional frameworks rather than modern clinical evidence, these ideas reflected a holistic understanding of the connection between food and wellness.

My own path into organ-based nutrition began over fifteen years ago. As both a scientist and a practitioner of traditional medicine, I was searching for ways to bridge the gap between ancient knowledge and modern health challenges. I learned that our ancestors prioritized organ meats because of their density of essential nutrients, and I wanted to understand how that applied today. As I explored this field more deeply, I also became aware of a growing concern: the quality of the foods we consume has changed, and not all organ meats available today reflect the purity or potency that our ancestors once relied on.

This realization sparked a deeper investigation into both the risks and the potential of modern organ therapy.

The Problem with Modern Organ Meats

While the historical use of organ meats reflects a deep respect for their nutritional value, the landscape has shifted. Modern industrial agriculture has introduced practices that have altered the quality of these once-sacred foods. Animals raised in confined feedlots are often exposed to antibiotics, synthetic hormones, and chemically treated feed. These inputs may not only affect the health of the animal but also the composition of the organs themselves.

Organs such as the liver and kidneys are biologically designed to filter and process compounds in the body. In conventionally raised animals, these organs may accumulate residues from medications, environmental toxins, or heavy metals. While regulatory systems exist to monitor food safety, concerns persist about the long-term effects of consuming organ meats from animals raised in unnatural or heavily medicated environments.

As awareness of these risks grows, more individuals are becoming mindful of where their food comes from and how it is produced. For those seeking the benefits of organ-based nutrition, the source and purity of the organs matter more than ever.

The Grass-Fed Revival

In response to growing concerns about food quality, a modern revival of ancestral eating practices has taken shape. At the center of this movement are grass-fed organ supplements, which offer a practical way to access the nutritional value of organs without the challenges of sourcing, preparing, or cooking them. These supplements are typically made by freeze-drying the organs of pasture-raised cattle and encapsulating the nutrient-rich powder for convenient use.

Grass-fed animals are raised on open pastures, allowed to graze naturally, and are not routinely exposed to antibiotics, growth hormones, or genetically modified feed. As a result, the organs from these animals retain their natural nutrient profiles, offering a cleaner and more consistent option for those seeking whole-food-based supplementation.

Liver, heart, kidney, spleen, and thyroid are among the most commonly used organs in supplement form, each valued for its unique nutrient density. For example, liver is a rich source of vitamin A, iron, and B12, while heart contains CoQ10 and essential amino acids. Kidney offers bioavailable selenium, and spleen is known for its naturally occurring heme iron and supportive peptides.

These supplements allow modern individuals to engage with the principles of whole-animal nutrition in a way that fits into busy lifestyles. For many, they represent a return to nutritional traditions that were once central to human health but have been largely forgotten in recent generations.

Although this book focuses on grass-fed beef organs, due to its accessibility, it is worth noting that other clean sources, such as porcine and ovine organs, are also available and used in specific supplement formulations. The most important factors remain consistent: purity, responsible sourcing, and respect for the nutritional complexity of each organ.

What to Expect in This Book

Now that we have explored the historical and cultural importance of organ consumption and the value of sourcing clean, grass-fed organ meats, we turn our attention to how these practices are being adapted in modern times. While ancient peoples consumed organs as part of a whole-animal diet, today we have access to grass-fed beef organ supplements that preserve this tradition in a convenient and accessible form. These supplements offer a way to reconnect with nutrient-dense foods without the need to prepare or cook organ meats.

In the chapters ahead, you will find detailed profiles of key organs that have become increasingly popular in the natural health community, including liver, heart, kidney, spleen, thyroid, and others. These supplements are valued for their rich concentration of naturally occurring vitamins, minerals, and compounds that contribute to overall nutritional support.

Here is what you can expect in each organ's profile:

Science-Informed Solution Benefits

Each organ supplement is introduced with a summary of its key nutrients and naturally occurring compounds. This includes a breakdown of essential vitamins, minerals, enzymes, and co-factors, along with a discussion of the body systems these nutrients are known to support. Insights are drawn from nutritional research, traditional practices, and scientific analysis of organ composition. This section is designed to offer educational context and does not make claims about treatment or guaranteed effects.

Customer-Reported Solution Benefits

To better understand how these supplements are being used in real life, we analyze patterns from thousands of user reviews. This section includes:

Use Case Patterns Observed

This highlights the most common reasons individuals report choosing a particular organ supplement. Based on recurring themes in user feedback, it reflects practical motivations such as energy support, cognitive clarity, metabolic balance, or immune resilience. It offers a glimpse into how people are incorporating these supplements into their routines.

Feedback Insights

This narrative summary captures how users describe their experiences with each organ, including the emotional and functional language they use. Whether users report feeling more focused, balanced, or energized, this section provides insight into the real-world sentiment behind their supplement use, in their own words.

Most Reported Benefits from Review Analysis

We provide a snapshot of the top benefits most frequently mentioned in verified customer reviews, using a percentage breakdown to illustrate which outcomes are most commonly noted. This helps clarify how these supplements are typically experienced and which benefits tend to stand out across a broad range of users.

This dual lens, one based on scientific understanding, the other on real-world experience, offers a well-rounded view of each organ's potential role in a modern wellness routine.

Reference Guide to Everyday Health Goals

At the end of the book, you will find a reference section that connects common wellness goals, such as immune support, energy, cognitive focus, or hormonal balance, with the organ supplements most often associated with those outcomes. This guide draws from both nutritional reasoning and user-reported feedback. It is intended as an educational tool and not as a replacement for personalized health care.

While this book focuses on grass-fed beef organs due to their accessibility and nutrient density, the principles of animal organ therapy can also apply to high-quality porcine and ovine organ supplements. Regardless of the source, purity and responsible sourcing remain essential.

This combined approach, merging ancestral wisdom, nutritional science, and modern consumer experience, aims to help you explore organ-based nutrition with clarity and confidence.

Beef Liver

Among the most respected nutrient-dense foods, grass-fed beef liver is widely regarded for its concentration of essential vitamins, minerals, and naturally occurring compounds. For generations, liver was considered one of the most valuable parts of the animal, often prioritized in traditional cultures for its ability to sustain strength and vitality. In many societies, it was consumed first after a hunt or reserved for individuals in need of dense nourishment, such as warriors, elders, or the ill. Today, freeze-dried liver supplements sourced from grass-fed cattle offer a modern way to access the same nutritional richness without the need for daily cooking or preparation.

Beef liver from pasture-raised animals is particularly notable for its content of bioavailable vitamin A, vitamin B12, iron, folate, and other supportive nutrients. These compounds occur in their naturally balanced form and are involved in a wide range of physiological functions, including red blood cell formation, energy metabolism, and cellular maintenance. Because the source animals graze on open pasture and are not routinely exposed to growth hormones, antibiotics, or chemically treated feed, grass-fed liver offers a clean and minimally processed supplement option for those seeking whole-food-based nutritional support.

Liver remains one of the most popular and widely used organ supplements available today. Its nutrient density, historical significance, and accessibility have made it a foundational choice for individuals interested in exploring animal organ therapy. Whether used on its own or combined with other organs in blended formulas, beef liver continues to play a central role in reconnecting modern wellness practices with time-honored nutritional traditions.

Science-Informed Beef Liver Benefits

Beef liver from grass-fed cattle is often described as one of the most nutrient-dense whole foods available. It contains a wide range of essential vitamins, minerals, and co-factors that play supportive roles in various physiological systems. Historically regarded as a foundational food across many cultures, liver's unique nutritional profile continues to attract attention for its potential to complement modern wellness routines.

Nutritional Support for Liver Function and Detoxification

The liver is a central organ in the body's metabolic system, responsible for processing nutrients and managing the breakdown of substances that enter the bloodstream. To carry out these complex processes efficiently, the liver depends on several key nutrients, many of which are found in abundance in beef liver. These include vitamin A, B12, folate, iron, and high-quality protein that provides essential amino acids.

Beef liver is a rich natural source of preformed vitamin A (retinol), which supports the liver's ability to regulate oxidative stress. It also contains compounds such as methionine and cysteine, which are precursors to glutathione, a compound often referred to as the body's master antioxidant. These nutrients contribute to the body's detoxification pathways by supporting enzyme systems involved in the neutralization and elimination of metabolic byproducts.

Another important compound found in beef liver is choline, which plays a key role in lipid metabolism. Choline supports the transport of fats from the liver, which helps maintain a healthy fat balance in the organ. Nutritional support from choline may be especially important in contexts where dietary fats are high or physical activity levels are low.

Support for Energy Metabolism and Nutrient Replenishment

Grass-fed beef liver contains several B vitamins, most notably B12, riboflavin, and folate, all of which are involved in the body's energy metabolism pathways. These nutrients help convert food into usable energy at the cellular level and assist in the formation of red blood cells, which are responsible for transporting oxygen throughout the body.

Because vitamin B12 and iron work together in oxygen delivery and mitochondrial energy production, beef liver is particularly helpful in supporting endurance and reducing feelings of fatigue due to nutritional depletion. For individuals with limited dietary intake of animal products, beef liver offers a concentrated source of these vital nutrients in a naturally occurring form.

Nutrient Support for Healthy Skin

One of the most well-known nutrients in beef liver is vitamin A in the form of retinol. This compound plays a key role in maintaining epithelial health, including skin structure and cell turnover. Adequate intake of vitamin A supports the skin's ability to regenerate and maintain a smooth, even appearance.

In addition to retinol, beef liver provides zinc, which contributes to tissue repair and the skin's natural barrier function. The synergy of these nutrients helps provide foundational support for individuals seeking to maintain skin clarity and resilience from the inside out.

Immune System Nutrient Support

Several compounds in beef liver contribute to the maintenance of a healthy immune response. Vitamin A is involved in the development of mucosal tissues, which serve as the first line of defense in both the respiratory and gastrointestinal systems. Iron and zinc, both found in bioavailable forms in beef liver, are important in the development and function of immune cells.

Copper, another trace mineral present in beef liver, supports the enzymatic systems involved in immune activity and oxidative stress regulation. By offering a broad spectrum of immune-related nutrients, beef liver can be considered a supportive addition to a nutrient-rich diet aimed at immune maintenance.

Cognitive and Neurological Nutrient Support

Beef liver contains key nutrients involved in brain and nervous system function. These include vitamin B12, folate, and choline. These compounds contribute to the synthesis of neurotransmitters, which are responsible for communication between brain cells, and support the maintenance of healthy nerve tissue.

Choline, in particular, is a precursor to acetylcholine, a neurotransmitter that plays a role in memory and learning. Additionally, the antioxidant content in liver may help the body manage oxidative stress, which has been associated with cognitive aging in scientific literature. These combined nutrients help support mental clarity and focus, especially when dietary intake of these compounds is limited.

Mood and Emotional Health Support

Beef liver contains nutrients associated with mood regulation, including B vitamins and iron. These nutrients play structural and functional roles in the synthesis of neurotransmitters such as serotonin and dopamine, which are involved in emotional regulation and psychological resilience.

While beef liver is not intended to replace medical or psychological treatment, its nutrient density may complement a whole-food-based approach to wellness for individuals seeking to support a balanced mood through nutrition.

Iron and Red Blood Cell Support

Beef liver is one of the richest dietary sources of heme iron, the form of iron that is most easily absorbed by the human body. It also contains vitamin B12 and folate, both of which work alongside iron in the production of red blood cells and the transportation of oxygen throughout the body.

Individuals who require additional support for maintaining healthy iron levels may benefit from including beef liver in their diet, particularly when seeking non-synthetic forms of supplementation.

Support for Hormonal and Thyroid Function

Beef liver offers nutrients that contribute to endocrine system function, including selenium, iron, vitamin A, and B vitamins. These compounds support the metabolic pathways involved in thyroid hormone conversion and adrenal system balance. Selenium, in particular, plays a role in the enzymatic activity needed for thyroid hormone activation.

By providing the nutrients required for endocrine signaling and energy regulation, beef liver supports the body's internal feedback systems in a balanced and natural way.

Customer-Reported Beef Liver Benefits

Grass-fed beef liver supplements have earned a strong reputation in the natural wellness community for their ability to nourish the body at a foundational level. With an impressive average rating of 4.6 out of 5 stars across thousands of verified reviews, they are frequently described as transformative, energizing, and essential. Many users refer to them as "a missing piece" or "a lifeline" in their healing journey. This enthusiasm reflects more than just satisfaction with a product. It reveals a deep sense of relief and restoration that users feel when their health begins to improve after years of fatigue, depletion, or frustration with conventional options.

The reviews we analyzed came from a wide range of individuals. Some were new parents navigating postpartum exhaustion, others were recovering from chronic stress or nutrient deficiencies, and many were trying to rebuild their energy and strength after major health setbacks. Despite these varied circumstances, one common thread connects them all. People often report that taking beef liver has helped them feel like themselves again, offering strength, vitality, and resilience that had previously felt out of reach.

Use Case Patterns Observed

Beef liver supplements are most often chosen by individuals seeking to improve energy, replenish low iron or ferritin levels, and overcome general fatigue. Many users begin their journey after struggling with traditional iron pills, which frequently caused nausea or offered little benefit. In contrast, beef liver is praised for being gentle on digestion while still delivering noticeable improvements in strength and stamina.

This supplement is especially popular among women addressing postpartum depletion, hormonal imbalances, or heavy menstrual cycles. Pregnant and breastfeeding users often mention that beef liver helped stabilize their energy levels and support a smoother recovery. Some women who had not responded well to synthetic vitamins found beef liver to be the first supplement that actually improved their mood, complexion, and sleep quality.

Beef liver is also frequently used by people recovering from long-standing nutritional deficiencies. Former vegans and vegetarians often turn to this supplement to rebuild nutrient stores that had been depleted over time. Individuals managing autoimmune conditions, histamine sensitivity, or thyroid challenges report using beef liver alongside kidney or thymus supplements as part of a broader healing routine.

Those following ketogenic, carnivore, or ancestral diets often use beef liver to enhance nutrient density without needing to consume cooked organ meats daily. Many users appreciate the convenience of capsules, especially when taste or lifestyle makes cooking liver impractical. Several reviewers also mention combining beef liver with bone marrow, adrenal, or collagen supplements to target specific wellness goals more effectively.

Feedback Insights

The emotional tone of these reviews is heartfelt and often deeply personal. Many users describe beef liver as "life-changing," "the best supplement I've ever taken," or "something I will never stop using." A large number of reviewers report feeling more energized, clear-headed, and emotionally stable, often within the first few days or weeks of use. One reviewer shared, "For the first time in years, I woke up feeling rested, and it brought tears to my eyes."

Physical improvements are frequently described with surprise and gratitude. Users mention stronger nails, glowing skin, new hair growth, and a clearer mind. Several people noted that family and friends began commenting on how much healthier and more vibrant they looked, which reinforced their belief that something meaningful was shifting in their bodies.

Mood and mental well-being are also recurring themes. Many individuals who had struggled with low mood, anxiety, or emotional exhaustion say they felt noticeably more balanced and grounded after starting beef liver. One woman described feeling like a "shell of herself" before trying the supplement and expressed joy at finally having the energy and calm needed to show up for her family. Others describe feeling more capable, more focused, and more resilient in the face of daily challenges.

While a few users experienced mild detox effects early on, such as temporary headaches or fatigue, most found that these passed quickly once they adjusted the dose.

Overall, the tone of these reviews is one of restoration and empowerment. Users describe beef liver not as a miracle, but as a steady source of real nourishment that helps the body perform the way it was meant to. It is not unusual to see phrases like "I feel like myself again," "this gave me my life back," or "finally something that works." These heartfelt responses suggest that beef liver is more than a supplement. For many, it is a turning point in their journey toward renewed health.

Most Reported Benefits from Review Analysis

To better understand how people experience beef liver supplements in real life, we examined thousands of verified reviews from users who reported positive outcomes. The chart below summarizes the most frequently mentioned benefits. The higher the percentage, the more commonly that benefit appeared in the feedback, giving you a data-informed perspective on what users tend to notice most when taking beef liver regularly.

For example, 36 percent of satisfied users described feeling a significant improvement in daily energy. This makes energy support the most commonly reported benefit of beef liver, often highlighted by users recovering from fatigue, nutrient depletion, or demanding routines.

Below is a summary table of beef liver's top benefits as reported by customers:

Benefit	%	Explanation
Energy Support	36%	Users frequently report feeling more energized, alert, and motivated throughout the day.
Hair Health	21%	Many mention noticeable improvements in hair thickness, strength, shine, and reduced shedding.
Skin Appearance	18%	Reviews often describe clearer, smoother, and more radiant skin, including reduced breakouts.
Nail Strength	15%	Users share that their nails became stronger, grew faster, and were less prone to breakage.
Reduced Fatigue	10%	Many note a decrease in overall tiredness and a greater ability to sustain energy throughout the day.

How to Use This Guide

If you are considering beef liver to support energy, skin health, or overall vitality, this data offers a helpful starting point. These percentages reflect how often each benefit was mentioned in positive reviews, and while individual results vary, they provide insight into the most commonly observed outcomes.

It is also worth noting that many reviewers describe experiencing more than one benefit at the same time. For example, a user who reports improved energy may also notice better skin clarity and stronger nails. In many cases, users share that the effects became more noticeable after consistent use over several weeks.

Beef liver supplements have received high praise across a wide range of health goals, and the consistency of these reports suggests they may serve as a valuable addition to many wellness routines.

Beef Thyroid

The thyroid gland plays a quiet but essential role in maintaining energy, metabolism, and overall balance within the body. When working optimally, it supports everything from temperature regulation to mental clarity and hormonal rhythm. Yet many people today face challenges related to low energy, sluggish metabolism, or feelings of imbalance, often without realizing that thyroid function may be a contributing factor.

Grass-fed beef thyroid supplements offer a natural way to nourish and support this vital gland. Derived from pasture-raised cattle and handled with care, these supplements provide naturally occurring thyroid nutrients, including bioavailable proteins, enzymes, and cofactors that are specific to thyroid tissue. By focusing on nutrient density and whole-food integrity, this form of organ support aligns with the traditional principle of "like supports like," in which consuming a healthy animal organ may help supply the building blocks needed for the same organ in the human body.

Whether you are seeking to maintain healthy energy levels, support metabolic wellness, or simply include more ancestral nourishment in your daily routine, grass-fed beef thyroid may offer a simple and targeted addition to your wellness toolkit.

Science-Informed Beef Thyroid Benefits

Grass-fed beef thyroid is valued for its ability to supply naturally occurring nutrients that help support the thyroid gland and its many roles in the body. This gland influences metabolism, energy, temperature regulation, and overall hormonal rhythm. The nutrients found in bovine thyroid tissue provide a unique combination of peptides, enzymes, and minerals that are highly specific to thyroid function. By focusing on whole-food nourishment rather than isolated compounds, grass-fed beef thyroid offers a traditional yet research-aligned way to support wellness in individuals looking to maintain thyroid health.

Supports Thyroid-Specific Nutritional Needs

The thyroid gland relies on a steady supply of nutrients to maintain its essential role in metabolic balance and energy regulation. Grass-fed beef thyroid contains naturally occurring forms of iodine and selenium, along with thyroid-specific proteins that may help the body meet these needs. Iodine is a foundational element required for the synthesis of thyroid hormones, while selenium supports the enzyme activity involved in hormone conversion processes. Providing these nutrients in a whole-food matrix allows for better compatibility with the body's natural mechanisms.

Incorporating beef thyroid into a supplement routine can be especially helpful for individuals who want to support their thyroid nutritionally, whether due to lifestyle stressors, environmental demands, or changes related to aging and metabolism.

Promotes Balanced Energy and Vitality

The thyroid gland plays a central role in how the body produces and uses energy. It influences how food is converted into fuel and how cells generate the energy needed for daily function. When thyroid support is lacking, people may experience feelings of low energy or find it difficult to maintain stamina. Grass-fed beef thyroid provides tissue-specific nutrients that are involved in energy metabolism, including compounds that help support mitochondrial function. Many individuals seeking to improve vitality choose beef thyroid supplements as a way to help restore balance and promote a steady sense of energy throughout the day.

Supports Healthy Metabolism and Weight Regulation

A balanced thyroid contributes to a healthy metabolism, helping the body use calories efficiently and regulate body weight. Nutrients found in grass-fed beef thyroid, such as iodine and tyrosine, play an important role in maintaining optimal metabolic activity. These compounds are naturally present in thyroid tissue and support the pathways involved in energy expenditure and nutrient utilization. Including thyroid-specific organ supplements may support individuals who are working toward better metabolic balance, especially when combined with a healthy diet and lifestyle.

Encourages Mental Clarity and Cognitive Focus

Thyroid health is closely linked to brain function. The hormones it helps regulate play an important role in maintaining cognitive sharpness, supporting neurotransmitter activity, and promoting mental clarity. Nutrient-rich beef thyroid supplements provide whole-food compounds that may help the body sustain these functions. Some individuals who experience mental fatigue, reduced concentration, or foggy thinking turn to thyroid-specific organ supplements for targeted nutritional support.

Contributes to Immune System Support

The immune system and thyroid gland share many regulatory pathways. When thyroid function is well supported, it can contribute to a more balanced immune response. Grass-fed beef thyroid contains peptides and cofactors that are naturally involved in the communication between the endocrine and immune systems. These compounds may help the body maintain stability during times of stress or seasonal change, especially for individuals looking to support immune resilience as part of their overall wellness plan.

Helps Maintain a Balanced Mood

The thyroid plays an influential role in how we feel, both physically and emotionally. When functioning optimally, it helps maintain stable levels of neurotransmitters that influence mood, outlook, and stress adaptation. Nutritional support from beef thyroid can offer foundational compounds the body may use to promote emotional steadiness and reduce the mental fatigue often associated with demanding schedules or hormonal changes. This makes thyroid-focused organ supplements a common choice for individuals seeking a natural way to help maintain emotional balance.

Supports Heart and Circulatory Health

Thyroid health has a well-established connection to cardiovascular wellness. It helps regulate heart rate, maintain blood vessel tone, and support cholesterol metabolism. Grass-fed beef thyroid contains nutrients that naturally align with these roles, offering a whole-food option for individuals looking to support cardiovascular balance through thyroid-related pathways. This type of organ support can be especially relevant for those seeking to nourish their heart and circulatory system as part of a broader self-care strategy.

Customer-Reported Beef Thyroid Benefits

Grass-fed beef thyroid supplements are gaining strong attention among individuals seeking to support energy, clarity, and overall well-being through nutrient-dense, organ-based nutrition. With an average customer satisfaction rating of 4.8 out of 5, users consistently describe feeling more balanced, energized, and focused after incorporating beef thyroid into their wellness routines.

Our analysis of real-world user experiences reveals powerful patterns in how this supplement is used and what types of changes people tend to report. While results can vary, a clear majority of reviewers noted benefits related to energy levels, mental sharpness, mood stability, and general vitality, especially among those navigating thyroid-related concerns.

This section summarizes common usage motivations and emotional feedback, based on verified reviews, to help you better understand how others are integrating grass-fed beef thyroid into their daily lives.

Use Case Patterns Observed

Beef thyroid supplements are most commonly chosen by individuals managing long-standing thyroid imbalances or seeking additional support for energy and metabolic health. Many reviewers are navigating subclinical thyroid conditions, hypothyroid symptoms, or have had challenges with prescription thyroid options. Others use beef thyroid alongside existing prescriptions to enhance their daily wellness routine.

A significant number of users mention using it after experiencing fatigue, weight management difficulties, mood fluctuations, or trouble with mental clarity. Some shared that they were able to transition from traditional thyroid medication under guidance, while others use it as complementary support. It is also popular among individuals with autoimmune thyroid conditions, as well as those pursuing a more holistic, food-based approach to hormonal balance.

In many cases, reviewers describe adding beef thyroid as part of a broader lifestyle shift that includes whole-food eating, stress reduction, and intentional supplementation. Dosing varies, with most people starting slowly and adjusting gradually, often in collaboration with a healthcare provider or personal research.

Feedback Insights

Across thousands of testimonials, users frequently express a deep sense of renewal and surprise at the positive changes they experienced. Phrases like "I feel like myself again," "the brain fog lifted," and "I have energy all day" appear often. Many describe noticeable improvements in the first few weeks, with energy, focus, and mood being the earliest changes reported.

One woman wrote that she had been taking thyroid medication for years but still felt fatigued and discouraged. After adding beef thyroid, she shared, "I finally feel clear-headed, energized, and stable. It's the first time in years I've felt this good." Another reviewer noted, "This supplement gave me back my motivation to move and work out, even after long days."

Several customers emphasized that their results improved over time and were grateful to have a natural option they could tolerate. Others were impressed by the emotional shift, saying things like, "I feel calm, steady, and more in control of my day," or "My anxiety disappeared, and I finally sleep through the night."

In addition to energy and mental clarity, many mentioned benefits such as improved hair and skin, more regular sleep, lighter mood, and less sensitivity to cold. Some reviewers mentioned that they now recommend the supplement to family members, clients, or health professionals because of how meaningful the changes have been.

This emotional tone, marked by gratitude, empowerment, and optimism, is one of the most consistent patterns in the feedback.

While experiences vary, the overwhelmingly positive sentiment reflects a strong sense of regained vitality and hope for ongoing improvement.

Most Reported Benefits from Review Analysis

To better understand how people experience the effects of beef thyroid, we analyzed thousands of customer reviews that described positive outcomes. The percentages shown in the table below reflect how often each benefit was mentioned by satisfied users. A higher percentage suggests that, among those who found the supplement helpful, that particular benefit stood out most.

For instance, 46% of reviewers referenced improvements in thyroid-related symptoms, suggesting this supplement may be particularly appreciated by those looking to support hormonal balance and metabolism. Others noted changes in energy, focus, and sleep quality, especially when used consistently as part of a daily routine.

Below is a summary of the most frequently reported benefits based on real-world experiences:

Benefit	%	Explanation
Thyroid Support	46%	Many users describe improvements in thyroid-related symptoms, including better hormonal balance, increased metabolic function, and an overall sense of well-being.
Energy Boost	28%	Users often report feeling more energized and less sluggish. Several describe greater stamina and a renewed ability to stay productive throughout the day.
Sleep Improvement	10%	Some reviewers noticed better sleep quality, with deeper rest and easier transitions into sleep, particularly when thyroid function felt more balanced.

Benefit	%	Explanation
Brain Fog Reduction	10%	A number of users mention feeling more mentally clear and focused, with reduced forgetfulness and sharper cognitive function.
Hair Health	7%	Several reviewers noted thicker, stronger hair and less shedding, particularly among those who had previously experienced thyroid-related hair thinning.

How to Use This Table

These percentages reflect the distribution of benefits reported in verified reviews from users who had a positive experience. While individual results vary, the data highlights what many people found most helpful. Some users noticed improvements in just one area, while others experienced a broader shift across multiple dimensions of wellness.

Combined with the supplement's strong overall rating of 4.8 out of 5, this feedback provides a valuable perspective on how beef thyroid may support key aspects of health such as thyroid balance, daily energy, mental clarity, sleep patterns, and hair vitality.

Beef Heart

Grass-fed beef heart is a nutrient-rich whole food that has long held a place in traditional diets, valued for its role in supporting vitality and resilience. Once reserved for those seeking strength and endurance, this organ meat is now available in supplement form, offering a convenient way to incorporate its nutritional benefits into modern life.

Beef heart provides a concentrated source of key nutrients, including Coenzyme Q10 (CoQ10), B vitamins, and high-quality protein. These compounds are involved in cellular energy production, cardiovascular support, and metabolic function. By nourishing the body at a foundational level, beef heart may help promote sustained energy and support heart health when used as part of a balanced routine.

Sourced from grass-fed, pasture-raised cattle, these supplements are produced without the use of hormones, antibiotics, or synthetic additives. For individuals seeking a food-based approach to wellness, beef heart offers a naturally derived option grounded in nutritional tradition and modern quality standards.

Science-Informed Beef Heart Benefits

Supports Cardiovascular Health

Beef heart is a naturally rich source of Coenzyme Q10 (CoQ10), a compound that plays a critical role in supporting heart function at the cellular level. CoQ10 contributes to energy production within heart muscle cells and helps reduce oxidative stress, which can otherwise affect cardiovascular resilience over time. By supplying this important nutrient through a whole-food source, beef heart offers nutritional support for those looking to promote cardiovascular wellness.

In addition to CoQ10, beef heart contains key B vitamins, especially vitamin B12, which are essential for the production of red blood cells and the delivery of oxygen throughout the body. Iron and zinc are also present, both of which help maintain balanced cholesterol levels and support vascular integrity. Together, these nutrients help sustain a healthy cardiovascular system when included as part of a balanced wellness approach.

This benefit is especially relevant for individuals seeking nutritional strategies to maintain cardiovascular vitality, manage age-related changes in heart function, or support healthy circulation.

Boosts Energy and Stamina

For those who experience occasional fatigue or dips in physical performance, beef heart provides foundational nutritional support. Its high content of CoQ10 enhances mitochondrial activity, which is essential for converting nutrients into usable energy at the cellular level. By supporting mitochondrial health, beef heart helps the body generate steady, sustained energy throughout the day.

The supplement also delivers bioavailable iron and complete protein, both of which are necessary for the production of red blood cells and the transportation of oxygen to tissues. These combined effects contribute to improved stamina, better recovery from physical activity, and overall vitality.

Individuals with demanding schedules, active lifestyles, or fatigue associated with nutritional gaps may find that beef heart offers meaningful support for energy and physical resilience.

Enhances Mental Clarity and Cognitive Health

Beef heart supports cognitive well-being through its unique blend of B vitamins, CoQ10, and iron. These nutrients help maintain proper neurological function by supporting neurotransmitter activity, reducing oxidative stress in brain tissue, and promoting healthy blood flow to the brain.

CoQ10 and B vitamins in particular are involved in mitochondrial function in brain cells, which helps sustain mental alertness and reduce occasional brain fog. When used consistently, beef heart may support sharper focus, improved clarity, and better cognitive performance during busy or mentally demanding periods.

This benefit is especially relevant for individuals seeking to support brain health through nutrition, whether due to age-related concerns, demanding cognitive tasks, or general focus and concentration challenges.

Promotes Immune Function and Recovery

The immune-supportive properties of beef heart are linked to its content of iron, zinc, and B vitamins. These nutrients are involved in the development and function of immune cells, helping the body respond to environmental stressors and maintain natural defenses. CoQ10 also plays a role in cellular repair and regeneration, which may support the body's recovery following physical exertion or stress.

For those recovering from illness or physical fatigue, or seeking to maintain immune strength during busy seasons, beef heart offers a nutrient-dense foundation for overall wellness and recovery support.

Customer-Reported Beef Heart Benefits

Beef heart supplements have received strong praise from thousands of users who describe noticeable improvements in energy, cardiovascular wellness, mood, and overall vitality. With an average satisfaction rating of 4.7 out of 5, this nutrient-rich organ supplement has gained popularity among those seeking a more natural way to support heart function, stamina, and circulation.

While each individual experience is unique, clear usage patterns and emotional feedback emerge from the reviews. Many users report adding beef heart to their routines when conventional approaches have left them with lingering fatigue, unstable blood pressure, or reduced endurance. Others highlight the supplement's role in helping them feel more grounded, energized, and resilient throughout the day.

By analyzing real-world experiences, we can better understand what people are actually using beef heart for, how they describe the effects, and which benefits are mentioned most frequently. These patterns offer a helpful glimpse into its potential role as part of a well-rounded wellness routine.

Use Case Patterns Observed

Most reviewers turn to beef heart for targeted cardiovascular support, particularly when dealing with elevated blood pressure, circulation issues, or a family history of heart concerns. A sizable group of users, ranging from seniors to athletes, take it specifically for improved stamina and daily energy. Many incorporate it as part of a larger wellness stack that includes other organ supplements to maximize nutrient intake and support overall metabolic health.

A number of individuals who previously experienced post-exercise fatigue, shortness of breath, or irregular heart rhythms mention noticeable improvements in those areas. Some chose beef heart for its naturally occurring CoQ10 content and report preferring it over synthetic versions. Additionally, reviewers often mention mental clarity and mood balance as unexpected yet welcome benefits, especially during periods of stress or seasonal emotional dips.

While many users take beef heart on its own, others combine it with liver, adrenal, or spleen supplements as part of a broader effort to support recovery, energy, and cardiovascular performance.

Feedback Insights

The emotional tone of customer feedback is overwhelmingly positive and often enthusiastic. Many reviewers express relief and gratitude after struggling with low energy, blood pressure fluctuations, or the side effects of medication. Phrases like "this gave me energy like I haven't felt in years," "I finally feel strong again," and "this is rocket fuel for my body" come up repeatedly, especially from older adults, athletes, and individuals recovering from stress or illness.

Others describe specific physical improvements, such as "my heart doesn't race on the stairs anymore," "no more daily headaches," and "I sleep more soundly now." Several reviewers note that they were skeptical at first but quickly became convinced by how their body responded. The words "grateful," "reliable," and "life-changing" are common, reflecting a strong emotional connection to the product's perceived benefits.

A few highlight the confidence they now feel in taking care of their heart health naturally, without relying solely on conventional approaches. This sense of empowerment and improved quality of life is a recurring theme across many reviews.

Most Reported Benefits from Review Analysis

Beef heart has earned a strong reputation as a nutrient-dense supplement that supports cardiovascular wellness, sustained energy, and physical stamina. With a consistently high satisfaction rating of 4.7 out of 5 stars, many users describe noticeable improvements in how they feel, particularly in areas related to heart function, circulation, and overall vitality.

To better understand what users most often experience, we analyzed thousands of reviews that shared positive feedback. The chart below reflects how frequently each benefit was mentioned among those satisfied users. A higher percentage indicates that the benefit was reported more often, offering a data-informed view of what Beef Heart is most commonly appreciated for.

For example, when 57 percent of positive reviews highlight heart health support, it suggests that many users observed improvements in how their heart and circulatory system felt after incorporating beef heart into their routine.

Below is a summary table of the top benefits users most often associate with Beef Heart:

Benefit	%	Explanation
Heart Health	57%	Many users report improved heart function, better circulation, and cardiovascular resilience. Some describe a greater sense of stability and stamina during physical activity.
Energy Boost	23%	A noticeable increase in daily energy. Users often mention feeling more awake, steady, and physically capable.

Benefit	%	Explanation
Blood Pressure	12%	Support for maintaining healthy blood pressure. Several reviewers observed more stable readings and reduced variability.
Stamina	5%	Enhanced physical stamina and ability to sustain effort throughout the day. This was especially noted by those with active lifestyles.
Endurance	4%	Greater resilience during exercise or demanding routines. Some users felt they could push further or recover more quickly.

How to Use This Guide

These reported patterns reflect the most common benefits mentioned in positive customer experiences. While individual results vary, the percentages shown can help you understand how others have used Beef Heart as part of their wellness journey.

It is also worth noting that many users report more than one benefit at a time, for example, improved energy often coincides with better stamina and cardiovascular support. In many cases, these effects became more apparent after several weeks of consistent use.

With high user satisfaction and a growing number of supportive reviews, Beef Heart continues to be valued as a foundational supplement for those seeking to nourish their cardiovascular system and build long-lasting energy and endurance.

Beef Kidney

Grass-fed beef kidney is a nutrient-rich organ supplement valued for its unique combination of vitamins, minerals, and naturally occurring compounds that help support foundational wellness. Historically incorporated into traditional diets around the world, kidney was often prized for its perceived ability to promote strength and overall vitality.

Today, grass-fed beef kidney supplements offer a convenient way to access these nutritional benefits without the need for cooking or preparation. They provide a natural source of B vitamins, selenium, zinc, and amino acids, nutrients known to play important roles in energy metabolism, immune support, and detoxification pathways. Because they are sourced from pasture-raised cattle and processed without synthetic additives, these supplements deliver a clean and holistic option for individuals seeking to nourish their bodies with ancestral foods.

Whether you are exploring nutrient-dense organ meats for the first time or looking to add kidney-specific support to your wellness routine, grass-fed beef kidney offers a traditional solution with modern accessibility.

Science-Informed Beef Kidney Benefits

Supports Histamine Breakdown and Digestive Sensitivity

Grass-fed beef kidney is valued for its naturally occurring diamine oxidase (DAO), an enzyme involved in breaking down excess histamine in the body. Elevated histamine levels can contribute to sensitivities such as occasional bloating, skin flushing, or digestive discomfort. For individuals who struggle with histamine overload or sensitivities to certain foods, beef kidney offers a unique dietary source of DAO to help support balance.

In addition to DAO, beef kidney contains essential nutrients like selenium and B vitamins, which are known to support a healthy intestinal lining and overall digestive function. These nutrients help maintain cellular integrity in the gut and assist in calming localized inflammation. For those looking to support histamine regulation and digestive well-being through nutrient-dense foods, beef kidney provides a traditional, science-supported option.

Nourishes and Supports Kidney Function

Beef kidney offers organ-specific nutrients that help support the health and function of the kidneys themselves. The kidneys play a central role in fluid balance, waste elimination, and the regulation of blood pressure and minerals. Grass-fed beef kidney contains selenium, B vitamins, and amino acids that contribute to these processes.

Selenium, in particular, acts as a powerful antioxidant that helps protect kidney tissues from oxidative stress, while B vitamins assist in energy metabolism and cellular repair. The protein and peptides naturally present in beef kidney also support tissue maintenance and regeneration. These properties make beef kidney a thoughtful addition to a wellness routine for those looking to maintain urinary and renal system support.

Supports Immune Resilience and Inflammatory Balance

Beef kidney is rich in selenium, zinc, and vitamin A, three nutrients with well-documented roles in immune function. Selenium helps regulate inflammation and oxidative stress at the cellular level, while zinc is essential for the development and activation of immune cells. Vitamin A supports the mucosal barriers in the gut and respiratory tract, which serve as the body's first line of defense.

Together, these nutrients help maintain a balanced immune response and support the body's ability to adapt to daily stressors. For individuals seeking to strengthen their immune defenses in a natural, food-based way, beef kidney offers a nutrient-rich option rooted in ancestral nutrition.

Promotes Natural Energy and Physical Vitality

The B vitamin content of beef kidney, particularly vitamin B12 and riboflavin, plays a critical role in supporting energy metabolism. These vitamins help convert dietary nutrients into usable cellular energy, which can be especially valuable for those experiencing occasional fatigue or low energy.

Combined with high-quality protein, these nutrients contribute to muscle recovery, endurance, and sustained physical activity. Beef kidney may benefit athletes, busy professionals, or anyone seeking to restore vitality without relying on synthetic energy boosters.

Provides Nutritional Support for Hormonal and Adrenal Balance

The adrenal glands, which help regulate the body's stress response, depend on a steady supply of nutrients like selenium, zinc, and certain amino acids. Grass-fed beef kidney contains these building blocks, which support the production and balance of adrenal hormones such as cortisol and aldosterone.

While beef kidney does not contain hormones itself, it offers precursors and cofactors that nourish the glands involved in hormonal regulation. Individuals managing stress-related fatigue or seeking to promote natural resilience may benefit from including beef kidney in their nutritional approach.

Supports Cardiovascular Health and Fluid Regulation

Because of the kidney's natural role in regulating minerals and hydration, beef kidney is rich in electrolytes such as potassium and sodium. These minerals help maintain proper fluid balance, nerve conduction, and healthy blood pressure regulation.

In combination with the antioxidant properties of selenium and vitamin A, these nutrients help support the vascular system and contribute to cardiovascular wellness. For those interested in natural ways to maintain circulatory and fluid balance, beef kidney offers a whole-food approach grounded in nutritional science.

Customer-Reported Beef Kidney Benefits

Thousands of individuals seeking to support their health naturally have turned to grass-fed beef kidney supplements, many of whom report striking changes in how their bodies respond to histamine, energy demands, and urinary wellness. With a 4.3 out of 5 overall rating, customer reviews point to notable improvements in histamine tolerance, inflammation management, energy levels, and kidney-related concerns. While experiences vary, recurring patterns in usage and feedback reveal how people are incorporating beef kidney into their wellness routines and what changes they most frequently notice.

Use Case Patterns Observed

Beef kidney supplements are most commonly used by individuals seeking support for histamine sensitivity, particularly those dealing with conditions like histamine intolerance, mast cell activation concerns, or frequent allergic reactions. Many users report years of trial and error with various remedies, including strict diets, multiple medications, and conventional antihistamines, often with limited or inconsistent results.

These supplements are also chosen by people aiming to restore kidney vitality, manage fluid retention, and promote urinary comfort. Some use beef kidney as part of a broader protocol that includes other beef organs like liver, thymus, or bone marrow, especially in support of immune health and adrenal balance. Additionally, a number of users begin with a low dose and slowly build up tolerance, particularly those who identify as highly sensitive to new supplements or organ products.

A smaller but meaningful segment of users incorporates beef kidney to support energy, mental clarity, and reduced systemic discomfort. These individuals often report overlapping concerns such as brain fog, fatigue, joint discomfort, and skin reactivity. In several cases, beef kidney is used alongside thyroid or adrenal supplements to target broader metabolic or hormonal imbalances.

Feedback Insights

Many reviewers express deep emotional relief and gratitude after discovering beef kidney, especially those who had felt exhausted by years of unexplained symptoms or food reactions. One user described the experience as "finally feeling like myself again," while another called it "a life-changing moment" after being able to eat a normal meal without symptoms. For many, histamine relief is the most dramatic shift, often marked by a reduction in hives, migraines, anxiety episodes, or facial flushing.

Several people highlight improved energy as a secondary but surprising benefit, with some describing it as "more drive to do things again" or "feeling restored for the first time in years." Emotional language around hope, gratitude, and even disbelief is common, particularly among users who had tried many other solutions without success. Some mention experiencing a "sense of calm" or "inner balance" shortly after beginning supplementation.

For those using the product to support kidney function directly, outcomes include less swelling in the legs or ankles, improved urine flow, and reduced water retention. One reviewer noted they were able to stop elevating their legs at night for the first time in years. Others speak of better sleep, clearer skin, and improved bowel regularity, benefits they often attribute to reduced internal inflammation or histamine load.

Importantly, many reviewers caution others to "go slow," especially those with sensitivities. Users frequently emphasize the importance of easing into a small dose, with some finding even a partial capsule enough to notice a difference. When the supplement works well, users often describe it not just as helpful but as essential, something they now rely on to maintain day-to-day stability.

Most Reported Benefits from Review Analysis

Beef kidney has become increasingly appreciated as a nutrient-dense supplement that may support kidney health, histamine regulation, and immune function. With an overall customer rating of 4.3 out of 5, thousands of users report noticeable improvements in areas such as urinary function, energy, and inflammation-related discomfort.

To better understand which benefits users most frequently experience, we analyzed a large sample of verified customer reviews. The table below reflects the percentage of positive reviews that mentioned each specific outcome. A higher percentage suggests that individuals with related goals or concerns may be more likely to notice similar results.

For example, if 44 percent of positive reviews mention kidney support, it highlights how often users associate this supplement with improved urinary wellness and detoxification.

Below is a summary table of beef kidney's top benefits as reported by customers.

Benefit	%	Explanation
Kidney support	44%	Many users describe improved urinary health, better fluid regulation, and support for overall kidney function. Some also note relief from chronic urinary discomfort.
Histamine balance	26%	Users managing histamine intolerance often report reduced congestion, skin irritation, and other histamine-related symptoms. Some attribute this to the natural presence of DAO enzymes.
Energy boost	16%	Increased daily energy and reduced fatigue are frequently mentioned. Users describe feeling more mentally alert and physically capable.
Inflammation control	7%	Some users report less joint stiffness, reduced swelling, and better post-activity recovery, contributing to greater comfort.
Immune support	6%	A smaller but consistent number of reviewers describe fewer seasonal illnesses and improved resilience to minor infections or colds.

How to Use This Guide

This benefit analysis is based on positive user experiences and is intended to offer insight into what people most often report. While individual results can vary, these patterns may help guide your decision if you are exploring support for kidney function, histamine balance, or overall vitality.

Many reviewers also noted that results became more noticeable with consistent use over several weeks. Some experienced multiple benefits simultaneously, such as improved energy and better digestion or enhanced circulation and reduced inflammation. When combined with a balanced lifestyle, beef kidney supplements appear to offer meaningful support for a range of wellness goals.

Beef Pancreas

Grass-fed beef pancreas is a naturally nutrient-rich organ supplement traditionally used to support digestive efficiency and metabolic wellness. In ancestral food traditions, the pancreas was often consumed for its role in maintaining energy balance and promoting digestive resilience, especially in those with demanding physical needs.

This organ is a natural source of digestive enzymes such as amylase, protease, and lipase, which help the body break down carbohydrates, proteins, and fats. It also provides important micronutrients like B vitamins, zinc, and selenium, which are involved in cellular energy production, antioxidant defense, and overall metabolic function. For individuals seeking to support healthy digestion or maintain steady energy throughout the day, grass-fed beef pancreas offers a food-based approach rooted in whole-animal nutrition. Sourced from pasture-raised cattle and produced without synthetic additives, this supplement reflects a clean and traditional way to nourish key physiological systems.

Science-Informed Beef Pancreas Benefits

Supports Blood Sugar and Metabolic Efficiency

Grass-fed beef pancreas naturally contains enzymes and micronutrients that contribute to healthy glucose metabolism. It provides amylase and lipase, two key digestive enzymes involved in breaking down carbohydrates and fats, which are essential for maintaining stable blood sugar levels and avoiding spikes or crashes in energy. The presence of zinc in beef pancreas is especially important, as this mineral plays a central role in the production and function of insulin, the hormone that regulates blood glucose.

When the body receives adequate enzymatic and nutritional support, it can metabolize macronutrients more efficiently, reducing strain on the pancreas and improving insulin sensitivity. For those looking to support blood sugar balance through dietary means, beef pancreas provides a concentrated source of nutrients that align with the body's natural metabolic functions.

Enhances Digestive Enzyme Activity and Nutrient Absorption

Beef pancreas is particularly rich in protease, amylase, and lipase, which assist in breaking down proteins, carbohydrates, and fats respectively. These enzymes are essential for proper digestion and the efficient absorption of nutrients. When digestive enzyme production is compromised, whether due to stress, age, or pancreatic insufficiency, nutrient breakdown and uptake may suffer, leading to symptoms such as bloating, gas, and fatigue.

By supplying the body with naturally occurring enzymes in a whole-food form, beef pancreas can complement the digestive process and reduce reliance on the body's own enzyme production. This may be especially beneficial for those with enzyme insufficiencies or individuals recovering from gastrointestinal stress. Supporting digestion in this way helps improve nutrient absorption and may contribute to reduced inflammation and better gut comfort over time.

Contributes to Pancreatic Tissue Health and Function

The pancreas serves a dual function as both an endocrine and exocrine organ, producing insulin and digestive enzymes. Grass-fed beef pancreas provides protein building blocks and micronutrients that contribute to the health and maintenance of this critical organ. Nutrients such as selenium and B vitamins are known to support antioxidant defenses and cellular repair mechanisms within pancreatic tissue.

Consuming beef pancreas may support the integrity of pancreatic cells by providing nutrients involved in energy metabolism, oxidative stress regulation, and enzyme production. While not a treatment, this organ-based support may help those seeking to reduce the overall burden on the pancreas or support its function nutritionally during periods of recovery or high metabolic demand.

Promotes Cellular Energy and Sustained Vitality

Grass-fed beef pancreas is a potent source of B vitamins, particularly B12 and riboflavin, which are essential for energy production at the cellular level. These vitamins help facilitate mitochondrial activity, the process by which cells convert food into usable energy. For individuals experiencing low energy, persistent fatigue, or symptoms of sluggish metabolism, these nutrients may provide the nutritional foundation for improved vitality.

By supporting stable blood sugar levels and enhancing nutrient absorption, beef pancreas also helps reduce fluctuations in energy that can occur after meals. Many individuals seek out this supplement to promote more consistent energy throughout the day, especially when managing metabolic stress or fatigue linked to blood sugar dysregulation.

Helps Maintain Immune Resilience and Reduces Inflammatory Stress

Beef pancreas contains selenium, zinc, and Vitamin A, nutrients known to play a vital role in supporting immune system function.

Selenium contributes to the activity of glutathione peroxidase, an important antioxidant enzyme, while zinc helps regulate immune cell signaling and promotes recovery from oxidative stress. Vitamin A supports the maintenance of mucosal barriers and overall immune surveillance.

When taken as part of a broader health routine, beef pancreas may support the body's natural defense systems and contribute to a more balanced inflammatory response. This is particularly valuable for individuals with long-standing inflammatory conditions or those who experience immune dysregulation due to nutrient depletion or chronic stress.

Supports Hormonal Regulation through Nutrient Cofactors

The pancreas is not only a digestive organ but also a major player in endocrine regulation, producing hormones that influence blood sugar, appetite, and metabolic rhythm. Zinc and selenium, both found in beef pancreas, are required cofactors in the synthesis and regulation of hormones such as insulin and glucagon.

Nutritional support for hormone production and signaling may be helpful for individuals managing metabolic imbalances, including those related to insulin sensitivity. By delivering these essential cofactors in their natural, food-based form, grass-fed beef pancreas offers a way to reinforce the body's hormonal framework and support homeostasis through diet.

Customer-Reported Beef Pancreas Benefits

Grass-fed beef pancreas has attracted attention among individuals looking for natural ways to support digestive health, energy, and metabolic balance. Based on real-world user feedback, this supplement has been praised for helping people who struggled with long-standing issues like bloating, sluggish digestion, post-meal fatigue, and blood sugar swings. Many reviewers had tried various enzyme products, restrictive diets, or conventional options with little success, only to find noticeable improvements after introducing beef pancreas into their routine. With an outstanding customer satisfaction rating of 4.6 out of 5, this supplement stands out as a supportive tool for those seeking gentle yet meaningful improvements in digestion and metabolic wellness.

Use Case Patterns Observed

Beef pancreas supplements were commonly used by individuals dealing with chronic digestive discomfort, including gas, bloating, constipation, sluggish bowel movements, and poor nutrient absorption. Several users mentioned long-standing digestive challenges including pancreatic insufficiency, or other metabolic imbalances that led them to search for enzyme support. A recurring pattern involved individuals feeling frustrated after trying standard enzyme blends, probiotics, or conventional approaches, only to turn to beef pancreas for a more bioavailable and food-based solution.

Others reported using the supplement to improve energy and reduce post-meal fatigue, especially when paired with high-protein or high-fat meals. A smaller group of reviewers also shared their use of beef pancreas to support blood sugar balance and hormonal fluctuations, particularly in connection with thyroid or adrenal fatigue. In some cases, pet owners reported positive results when using beef pancreas to support digestive recovery in animals, especially dogs with pancreatic or malabsorption issues.

Feedback Insights

Many reviewers expressed a sense of deep relief and gratitude, noting that beef pancreas offered them the first meaningful improvements they had experienced in years. Words like "finally," "amazing," and "life-changing" came up frequently, especially among those who had struggled with frustrating cycles of trial and error.

Users described feeling "lighter," "clear-headed," and "energized," often noticing better digestion with fewer side effects like bloating, reflux, or intestinal discomfort. One common theme was the emotional shift that occurred when digestion improved. Several people shared that better gut function led to improved mood, less anxiety, and more consistent energy throughout the day.

Multiple users noted that they were able to reduce or stop other digestive aids they had relied on, such as probiotics, over-the-counter enzyme capsules, or antacids. Reviewers often reflected on how taking beef pancreas helped restore a sense of normalcy in daily life, such as waking up with more energy, enjoying meals without discomfort, or feeling mentally focused again. Even among those who started the supplement skeptically, many reported being surprised by the steady and noticeable improvements over time.

Most Reported Benefits from Review Analysis

Beef pancreas supplements are often chosen by individuals seeking natural support for digestive comfort, enzyme function, and overall gut health. With a customer rating of 4.6 out of 5 across thousands of reviews, many users describe noticeable changes in how their body processes food, from reduced bloating and gas to improved nutrient absorption and energy.

Our analysis of verified positive reviews highlights which outcomes were most frequently mentioned by users who experienced benefits. These percentages reflect how often a particular improvement came up among those satisfied with the supplement. A higher percentage means that more users reported seeing that result in their daily lives.

For instance, if 27 percent of users mentioned better stomach support, it indicates a trend among those who found relief from discomfort, reflux, or sluggish digestion. These data points can help you anticipate what kinds of benefits others have experienced when using beef pancreas as part of their wellness routine.

Below is a summary table of beef pancreas's top benefits as reported by customers:

Benefit	%	Explanation
Stomach Support	27%	Many users reported relief from discomfort, sensitivity, or acid imbalance, often noting easier digestion after meals.
Pancreas Support	21%	Users experienced improved enzyme activity, helping them break down proteins, fats, and carbs more effectively.
Gut Health	20%	Customers frequently mentioned better gut function, fewer disruptions, and improved digestive regularity.
Digestion Support	19%	Many noticed overall smoother digestion, with less fatigue after meals and better nutrient uptake.
Bloating Relief	13%	A significant number of reviewers experienced less bloating, pressure, and abdominal gas throughout the day.

How to Use This Table

This table is designed to help you quickly understand what others have most commonly experienced when taking beef pancreas supplements. While everyone's body responds differently, the percentages shown reflect patterns reported by real users who shared positive outcomes.

If you are looking for support with digestive discomfort, enzyme activity, or overall gut function, consider starting with the benefits most frequently reported, such as stomach support or pancreatic function. These are not guaranteed effects, but they give you a helpful sense of how the supplement may align with your needs based on collective feedback.

Use this as a practical reference, not a promise. Your experience may differ depending on your body, health status, and how consistently you use the supplement. The goal is to support your wellness journey with realistic expectations grounded in actual user insight.

Beef Organs Blend

The grass-fed beef organs blend is a comprehensive blend of five nutrient-dense organs: liver, heart, kidney, pancreas, and spleen. Long valued in traditional diets, these organs are rich in naturally occurring vitamins, minerals, peptides, enzymes, and co-factors that work synergistically to support overall health and vitality.

Each organ contributes unique nutritional properties. Liver is a concentrated source of essential nutrients that help support energy metabolism and foundational wellness. Heart supplies naturally occurring compounds like CoQ10 and B vitamins associated with cardiovascular and cellular energy support. Kidney provides peptides and enzymes that may assist with immune modulation and nutrient filtration. Pancreas contains enzymes that aid in the breakdown of macronutrients and support digestive processes. Spleen is a source of heme iron and bioavailable nutrients involved in red blood cell support and immune readiness.

Sourced from grass-fed, pasture-raised cattle and processed without synthetic additives, this supplement offers a traditional, food-based way to provide foundational nourishment across multiple systems of the body.

Science-Informed Beef Organs Blend Benefits

Supports Whole-Body Nutritional Balance

Beef Organs Blend delivers a concentrated combination of nutrients derived from five distinct organs: liver, heart, kidney, pancreas, and spleen. This whole-food supplement provides naturally occurring vitamins A, B12, D, and K2, along with essential minerals like iron, zinc, selenium, and copper. These nutrients are presented in their bioavailable forms, making them readily absorbable and usable by the body. The synergy between these organs helps support a broad range of physiological functions including energy metabolism, immune defense, detoxification, cardiovascular balance, and digestive efficiency. This comprehensive approach offers foundational support for multiple body systems, making it a uniquely integrative supplement choice.

Promotes Cellular Energy and Vitality

Liver, heart, and kidney are particularly rich in nutrients that are vital for cellular energy production. Vitamin B12 and heme iron from these organs support the formation of red blood cells and oxygen transport throughout the body. Coenzyme Q10, found naturally in heart tissue, plays a central role in mitochondrial function, which is essential for sustained physical and mental energy. By delivering these nutrients in food-based form, the Organs Blend may help reduce feelings of fatigue, enhance daily stamina, and support those with nutrient-related low energy states.

Supports a Balanced Immune Response

Spleen and liver tissues are dense sources of bioavailable compounds that contribute to healthy immune system regulation. The spleen contains naturally occurring peptides and cofactors involved in immune cell development and antibody production. Liver contributes key nutrients such as retinol (preformed vitamin A), which is critical for the integrity of mucosal barriers and immune signaling. Zinc and selenium, present in both kidney and pancreas tissues, play supportive roles in cellular repair and antioxidant protection. Together, these nutrients may promote immune readiness and help maintain a balanced response to internal and external stressors.

Encourages Cardiovascular and Circulatory Wellness

Heart and kidney organs contain nutrients and compounds that contribute to cardiovascular health. Heart tissue is a natural source of CoQ10, which plays a vital role in supporting energy production in cardiac muscle and may assist in maintaining healthy blood pressure. Kidney tissue provides electrolytes such as potassium and sodium that are essential for fluid balance, vascular tone, and overall circulatory function. This combination may offer targeted support for maintaining healthy cardiovascular rhythm and blood flow.

Aids Digestion and Nutrient Assimilation

Pancreas tissue contributes naturally occurring digestive enzymes including amylase, protease, and lipase. These enzymes help break down carbohydrates, proteins, and fats, improving digestive efficiency and nutrient absorption. By supporting the body's own enzymatic activity, beef pancreas may help alleviate occasional bloating, discomfort, or sluggish digestion. Additionally, the pancreas plays a role in glucose metabolism, and the compounds it contains may contribute to maintaining healthy blood sugar balance in those with mild metabolic challenges.

Supports Hormonal Health and Stress Regulation

Liver and kidney are sources of essential cofactors that support the endocrine system. Zinc and selenium help facilitate thyroid hormone activation, while nutrients found in kidney tissue may aid adrenal hormone balance. These organs contribute compounds that help regulate the body's response to physical and emotional stress, supporting cortisol balance and helping the body recover from daily challenges. This benefit may be particularly relevant for those managing fatigue or hormonal fluctuations associated with lifestyle stress or nutritional deficiencies.

Encourages Detoxification and Blood Cell Support

Liver and spleen work together to support natural detoxification and red blood cell maintenance. The liver is the body's central organ for neutralizing toxins, metabolizing hormones, and processing environmental compounds. It also contributes to the conversion and activation of several nutrients. The spleen helps recycle iron and supports the balance and function of red and white blood cells. The nutrients found in these organs may assist the body in maintaining healthy detoxification pathways and robust blood health over time.

Customer-Reported Beef Organs Blend Benefits

Beef Organs Blend supplements have gained strong support from users seeking a natural, whole-food-based way to restore energy, improve nutrient intake, and support multiple systems at once. With an average rating of 4.6 out of 5 stars, thousands of users have shared experiences highlighting how this multi-organ formula may help with energy, hormonal balance, skin appearance, digestive comfort, and general vitality. These reports come from individuals with a wide range of backgrounds and health goals, especially those looking to nourish their bodies with nutrient-rich organ blends without needing to prepare and consume fresh organ meats. While experiences vary, many customers report consistent and noticeable improvements after regular use. The following insights reflect common use patterns and emotional responses shared by satisfied users.

Use Case Patterns Observed

Beef Organs Blend is widely chosen by individuals seeking comprehensive daily nourishment, especially when dealing with low energy, hormonal shifts, or feelings of nutritional depletion. It is often turned to by those who feel they've "tried everything" and are looking for a more natural, food-based way to restore vitality and balance. This blend is particularly popular among people following ancestral, carnivore, or ketogenic lifestyles, as well as those wanting a simpler alternative to synthetic multivitamins or isolated nutrients. Many users incorporate it as a foundational supplement to support overall wellness, often combining it with other targeted organ capsules, like liver, marrow, or adrenal, for a more personalized approach.

Feedback Insights

Customers frequently describe a transformative shift in how they feel after taking Beef Organs Blend, with many reporting changes that they describe as "life-giving," "energizing," or "profound." One of the most consistent themes is the emotional relief users feel when they regain a sense of vitality after years of exhaustion, particularly for women managing hormonal imbalances, menstrual discomfort, or postpartum symptoms. Many reviews express a deep gratitude, with users stating that the supplement helped them "feel like themselves again" or brought back a sense of normalcy they hadn't experienced in years. Energy improvements are described as stable and sustainable rather than jittery or artificial. Others note enhanced mood stability, better sleep, reduced brain fog, and even unexpected benefits such as shinier hair or clearer skin. Several users mention initial detox symptoms that resolved with dosage adjustment, and many emphasize that they experienced results faster than expected, sometimes within days. Despite the capsule size or taste being mentioned occasionally, most consider the benefits to far outweigh any minor inconvenience. A strong undercurrent of hope, relief, and empowerment runs through these reviews, especially among those who had felt overlooked or dismissed in traditional healthcare settings.

Most Reported Benefits from Review Analysis

Beef Organs Blend is widely appreciated by users looking to support their energy, skin, and overall vitality through a whole-food, nutrient-rich approach. With an average rating of 4.6 out of 5 stars across thousands of reviews, this multi-organ supplement has generated a high level of user satisfaction, particularly among those who are seeking a natural way to improve how they feel on a daily basis.

Our analysis of thousands of positive reviews shows which benefits users report most often. The percentages below reflect how frequently each benefit was mentioned among those who shared favorable experiences. These figures do not guarantee individual outcomes but can provide helpful guidance based on real-world patterns. If a particular benefit is frequently reported, it may be more likely to reflect the kinds of support people notice when taking this supplement regularly.

For example, if 53 percent of positive reviews mention increased energy, that suggests a strong trend among users experiencing greater stamina, reduced fatigue, and better day-to-day functioning.

Below is a summary table of beef organs blend's top benefits as reported by customers:

Benefit	%	Explanation
Energy boost	53%	Many users report a noticeable improvement in energy, stamina, and daily drive, often describing a return of vitality.
Skin health	22%	Users frequently mention clearer, more hydrated skin and a healthier overall appearance. Some noted improvements in acne or dryness.
Hair health	12%	Several reviews highlight stronger, shinier, and thicker hair, especially among those with previous thinning or hair loss.
Fatigue reduction	9%	Many users who experienced chronic fatigue describe feeling more balanced and capable throughout the day.
Immune support	5%	A smaller but meaningful number of users report fewer seasonal issues and a general sense of increased resilience.

How to Use This Table

This table highlights the most commonly reported benefits based on thousands of verified customer reviews. The percentages indicate how often a specific benefit was mentioned among users who had a positive experience with Beef Organs Blend. These figures do not suggest guaranteed results, but they can provide helpful context as you consider whether this supplement aligns with your personal wellness goals.

If you are primarily seeking more energy or resilience against fatigue, it may be helpful to note that over half of users who saw positive results mentioned increased energy. Similarly, if you are exploring support for hair or skin health, many reviewers reported improvements in these areas as well. This can guide your expectations and help you track your own progress over time.

As always, individual results vary. Some people may notice changes within a few days or weeks, while others may take longer depending on their baseline nutrient levels, lifestyle, and health status. Listening to your body, starting with a low dose, and being consistent are all important parts of the process.

Beef Colostrum

Beef colostrum is a nutrient-dense substance collected from the first milk of pasture-raised cows after giving birth. Traditionally regarded as one of nature's most complete and vitalizing foods, colostrum contains a concentrated profile of compounds that contribute to early-life immune defense and tissue development. When taken as a supplement, it offers a wide range of health-supportive properties that can benefit adults seeking foundational support for resilience and recovery.

Sourced from grass-fed, pasture-raised cattle, beef colostrum provides immunoglobulins, lactoferrin, growth factors, and essential nutrients that support immune system balance, gut lining integrity, and cellular repair. Its bioactive compounds are known to work synergistically to maintain a healthy internal environment and help the body respond more effectively to stressors. For individuals seeking natural options to promote vitality, digestive comfort, and immune readiness, beef colostrum remains a time-tested and comprehensive choice.

Science-Informed Beef Colostrum Benefits

Supports Immune Health and Natural Resilience

Beef colostrum provides a rich source of bioactive compounds that help maintain immune system balance. It contains naturally occurring immunoglobulins (such as IgG, IgA, and IgM), lactoferrin, and proline-rich polypeptides (PRPs), which contribute to immune modulation and defense. These components help bind and neutralize environmental stressors, supporting the body's natural ability to defend against unwanted organisms and maintain immune readiness. For individuals seeking broader support during periods of seasonal or environmental challenges, colostrum offers a natural and nutrient-dense option.

Helps Maintain Gut Integrity and Digestive Comfort

Colostrum is a valuable source of growth factors, including insulin-like growth factor 1 (IGF-1) and epithelial growth factor (EGF), which help maintain the structural integrity of the intestinal lining. These compounds have been studied for their potential to support mucosal barrier function and promote gastrointestinal tissue maintenance. In addition, colostrum's immunoglobulins assist in binding unwanted microbes and promoting a more balanced internal environment. Together, these actions help support digestive wellness, nutrient absorption, and gut comfort for those managing everyday gastrointestinal stress.

Provides Nutritional Support for Physical Recovery

The naturally occurring compounds in beef colostrum may support recovery from physical exertion by helping the body maintain healthy muscle tissue and reduce oxidative stress. Growth factors found in colostrum are known to influence cellular regeneration and may contribute to tissue resilience following exercise or physical strain. This makes colostrum a suitable addition for individuals who engage in regular training or those looking for nutritional support after physical activity.

Promotes Normal Inflammatory Balance and Tissue Health

Colostrum contains compounds such as lactoferrin and immunoglobulins that help regulate inflammatory responses and support the body's natural healing processes. These bioactive nutrients are involved in maintaining cellular communication and supporting healthy tissue repair mechanisms. Many individuals turn to colostrum as part of their overall strategy to maintain joint function, skin integrity, and recovery from routine wear and tear.

Supports Healthy Aging and Vitality

Beef colostrum provides a broad array of nutrients that may support cellular health over time. Its growth factors, antioxidant peptides, and essential proteins contribute to foundational wellness by promoting regeneration, reducing environmental oxidative stress, and helping the body maintain strength and resilience. As part of a daily health regimen, colostrum may support vitality and well-being across all stages of life.

Customer-Reported Beef Colostrum Benefits

Beef colostrum has earned consistent praise from users who describe it as one of the most impactful supplements they've tried. With an average rating of 4.5 out of 5 stars across thousands of reviews, many individuals report meaningful improvements in gut function, immune resilience, energy, and skin clarity. While results naturally vary, this feedback highlights the broad range of wellness goals that colostrum may help support.

Unlike isolated vitamins, beef colostrum is a whole-food-based supplement packed with naturally occurring compounds such as immunoglobulins, growth factors, and enzymes. These nutrients may explain why users consistently describe a noticeable difference in how they feel, often within just a few weeks of use. In our analysis of reviews, people commonly mention improvements in digestion, vitality, mood, and skin tone, making it a popular choice for both long-term health support and targeted wellness goals.

The following summary reflects the real-world patterns emerging from verified customers with positive experiences. While individual responses vary, this section can help you better understand what people most frequently report, how they use colostrum, and the kinds of outcomes they describe.

Use Case Patterns Observed

Beef colostrum is often selected by individuals looking for comprehensive internal support, especially in cases involving gut discomfort, immune challenges, skin conditions, or fatigue. Many users report turning to colostrum after years of digestive distress, food sensitivity, or inflammation-related discomfort, including those managing autoimmune issues. Several reviewers mention trying it as a follow-up to conventional care or after standard approaches failed to deliver results.

Others are drawn to colostrum for its potential to support resilience and recovery. Athletes and highly active individuals describe using it to improve stamina, accelerate workout recovery, and maintain consistent energy. A subset of users report turning to colostrum to improve skin elasticity, reduce puffiness, or address flare-ups associated with dietary triggers or stress. Some parents also share that they've used colostrum for children experiencing eczema, food intolerance, or immune sensitivity.

The most commonly observed pattern is multi-purpose use: many reviewers describe colostrum as a foundation for gut health that simultaneously enhances immunity, improves energy levels, and boosts skin appearance. It is often used alongside other organ-based supplements for broader wellness benefits.

Feedback Insights

Customer reviews reflect a high level of satisfaction, with many describing colostrum in deeply appreciative terms. One user called it "my #1 be-all, end-all" and credited it with improvements in digestion, mood, energy, and skin tone. Others echoed this, sharing how they felt "calmer, clearer, and more balanced" after just a few weeks. Reviewers frequently mention long-standing health frustrations that began to shift once colostrum became part of their routine.

Gut-related relief is one of the most cited benefits. People mention reduced bloating, improved bowel regularity, and a return to eating foods they had previously avoided. One reviewer noted that after 20 years of digestive challenges, they were finally able to reintroduce foods without discomfort. Others spoke of "a calm stomach" or described colostrum as "the only thing that worked" after trying many different approaches.

Energy and stamina are also frequently highlighted. Some reviewers report feeling more energized during the day, even with demanding work or intense physical activity. One user described it as "a wow factor for my workouts," while others shared how they now feel more motivated, focused, or emotionally even. Several mentioned better sleep quality and waking up feeling refreshed.

Skin improvements are another key area of feedback. Many describe clearer, brighter, or more hydrated skin, with fewer flare-ups. Several individuals noted that friends or family asked what they were doing differently based on visible changes.

In addition to the physical effects, many users express appreciation for the company's integrity and support. Dozens of reviews mention responsive communication and personalized guidance from the founder, which seems to have built a sense of trust and community among customers. This connection adds emotional weight to their testimonials, with many users sharing that they felt "heard," "guided," or even "healing with hope again."

Most Reported Benefits from Review Analysis

Beef colostrum has earned consistent praise from users for its broad wellness support, particularly in the areas of gut health, energy, and skin vitality. With an average customer rating of 4.5 out of 5 stars, many people describe it as a foundational supplement that helped them feel more balanced, resilient, and energized.

We analyzed thousands of positive reviews to identify the benefits users most frequently experienced. The percentages below reflect how often each benefit was mentioned by reviewers who had favorable results. While everyone responds differently, these figures can offer a helpful starting point when considering whether beef colostrum aligns with your health goals.

For example, if 25 percent of reviewers mentioned improvements in gut health, it suggests that individuals with digestive concerns were more likely to report noticeable relief in this area.

Below is a summary of the top benefits people report after using beef colostrum:

Benefit	%	Explanation
Gut health	25%	Many users report improvements in digestion, less bloating, and a stronger, more balanced gut.
Energy boost	25%	A noticeable increase in daily stamina, alertness, and reduced feelings of fatigue.
Skin health	22%	Clearer, more hydrated skin with fewer flare-ups or irritations, according to user feedback.

Benefit	%	Explanation
Immune support	16%	A stronger immune response, with fewer seasonal challenges and an overall sense of resilience.
Digestion support	12%	Easier digestion and better nutrient absorption, with less discomfort after meals.

How to Use This Table

This table offers a quick reference to help you understand what real users report most often when using beef colostrum. It does not predict individual results or offer medical advice, but it highlights trends in positive experiences that may align with your own needs. If you are exploring colostrum to support digestion, boost your energy, or improve skin clarity, these insights can help you prioritize which outcomes to monitor as you begin your own journey.

While percentages reflect user patterns, remember that everyone's health profile is different. The best way to evaluate this supplement is to start slowly, observe how your body responds, and track the outcomes that matter most to you.

Beef Bone and Marrow

Beef bone and marrow from grass-fed, pasture-raised cattle have long been valued in traditional nutrition for their rich nutrient profile and foundational role in whole-body wellness. Today, these time-honored foods are making a strong return as concentrated supplements, offering a natural source of support for those looking to nourish their bodies from within.

Bone and marrow are abundant in essential nutrients such as collagen, calcium, phosphorus, and beneficial fats including omega-3s. These elements are naturally found in forms the body can recognize and absorb, making beef bone and marrow a practical choice for those seeking to support joint function, skeletal strength, immune health, and overall vitality. By integrating these nutrient-dense components into modern wellness routines, many individuals are rediscovering the deep nourishment once central to ancestral diets.

Science-Informed Beef Bone and Marrow Benefits

Supports Bone Strength and Structural Integrity

Beef bone and marrow provide a concentrated source of foundational minerals including calcium, phosphorus, and magnesium, which are essential for building and maintaining strong skeletal structure. These minerals work synergistically to support bone mineralization, helping to maintain density and reduce the risk of age-related bone loss.

In addition, bone contains naturally occurring collagen, a structural protein that enhances the resilience and flexibility of the bone matrix. Collagen helps reduce brittleness and supports the internal scaffolding that gives bones their strength and ability to withstand stress. These combined elements make beef bone and marrow a practical option for individuals seeking to nourish bone tissue and support long-term skeletal health.

Promotes Joint Comfort and Mobility

Beef bone and marrow are rich in compounds that play a direct role in joint health, including naturally occurring collagen, gelatin, glucosamine, and chondroitin. Collagen and gelatin contribute to the strength and elasticity of connective tissues, supporting joint cushioning and mobility. Glucosamine and chondroitin, both naturally present in cartilage and marrow, are involved in maintaining joint lubrication and structural integrity.

By supporting the structural framework of cartilage and promoting the repair of connective tissue, these nutrients help reduce mechanical stiffness and support comfortable movement. These effects are especially valued by individuals experiencing joint discomfort, athletes, or those seeking to maintain mobility with age.

Supports a Balanced Immune Response

Beef marrow contains immune-supportive micronutrients such as zinc, selenium, vitamin A, and vitamin D, which play key roles in regulating the body's defense systems. Zinc and selenium act as cofactors in antioxidant enzymes that help neutralize oxidative stress, while vitamins A and D are involved in the modulation of both innate and adaptive immune responses.

Additionally, the healthy fats and lipids found in marrow help transport fat-soluble nutrients and support cellular health. Together, these compounds contribute to a nourished immune environment that is better equipped to respond to everyday challenges while maintaining internal balance.

Nourishes Skin, Hair, and Nail Health

The collagen and gelatin found in beef bone and marrow also play a key role in the health of skin and other connective tissues. Collagen contributes to skin elasticity and hydration by supporting the extracellular matrix, while gelatin supplies the amino acids needed for tissue regeneration.

Many individuals seek out collagen-rich foods to help maintain the appearance of firm, smooth skin and to support the strength and growth of hair and nails. Regular intake of collagen from food-based sources such as beef bone and marrow may be a helpful part of a broader approach to healthy aging and personal care.

Promotes Gut Lining Integrity and Digestive Support

Gelatin, a key component of bone-derived nutrients, is known for its ability to bind water and support the protective mucus layer of the gut. This can help soothe the digestive tract and support the body's natural efforts to maintain intestinal lining integrity. These effects are especially relevant for individuals navigating occasional digestive discomfort or seeking to promote gut balance.

In addition, the amino acids present in bone and marrow, such as glycine and glutamine, play important roles in gut wall repair, enzyme production, and nutrient transport. These functions help support digestion, absorption, and microbial balance throughout the gastrointestinal tract.

Contributes to Energy Metabolism and Vitality

Beef bone and marrow naturally supply B vitamins, essential fatty acids, and other micronutrients that support mitochondrial energy production. B vitamins, particularly B12 and riboflavin, are involved in the conversion of carbohydrates, fats, and proteins into usable cellular energy.

Meanwhile, the healthy fats found in marrow can serve as a slow-burning energy source that supports endurance and metabolic stability. These properties make bone and marrow supplements a practical nutritional addition for individuals experiencing physical fatigue or recovering from physical stress, illness, or nutrient depletion.

Customer-Reported Beef Bone and Marrow Benefits

Beef bone and marrow supplements have become a trusted resource for individuals seeking deeper nourishment, particularly those looking to support joint comfort, bone strength, vitality, and recovery. Across thousands of reviews, users consistently report noticeable improvements in their mobility, energy levels, mood, skin appearance, and overall sense of well-being. With an average customer rating of 4.5 out of 5 stars, these whole-food supplements have earned a place in the wellness routines of people dealing with everything from recovery fatigue to daily joint discomfort.

While benefits vary from person to person, our analysis reveals distinct patterns in how people are using beef bone and marrow, and what kinds of changes they report most often. The following insights are drawn from verified reviews that specifically mention positive effects attributed to bone and marrow support, giving you a clearer picture of what to expect.

Use Case Patterns Observed

Many individuals turn to beef bone and marrow supplements during times of physical recovery, stress, or chronic nutrient depletion. Users describe using these capsules to complement an animal-based diet, aid recovery from surgery or joint issues, or enhance a whole-body healing regimen that includes liver, kidney, and other organ support. Others mention adding bone and marrow to their routine after experiencing nutrient imbalances, hair thinning, gum issues, or prolonged fatigue.

A noticeable group of users includes individuals recovering from long-standing health burdens, such as chronic digestive issues, injury, or autoimmune challenges, who report seeking a more bioavailable form of foundational nourishment. For those already familiar with collagen or bone broth, bone and marrow capsules are often viewed as a concentrated, travel-friendly upgrade. They are also a popular addition to supplement stacks targeting joint function, skin rejuvenation, and vitality restoration.

Feedback Insights

Emotionally, the feedback is rich with gratitude, relief, and surprise. Many users say they were "shocked" by how quickly they noticed positive changes in energy, mobility, or skin tone, often within just a few days of use. Several describe bone and marrow as "deeply nourishing," giving them a calm, stable energy that helped them power through daily tasks or resume exercise routines they had long put on hold.

Common phrases include: "I feel like myself again.", "I didn't realize how depleted I was until I felt the difference.", "My joints move more freely, and I can walk without thinking about pain.", "My skin and hair look better than they have in years.", "This gave me hope when nothing else helped."

Reviewers who previously experienced detox symptoms with other organ supplements often report that bone and marrow felt more stabilizing and easier to tolerate over time. Others express a sense of empowerment, noting that the product helped them reconnect with a sense of strength and resilience they hadn't felt in a long time.

Most Reported Benefits from Review Analysis

Beef bone and marrow has received widespread appreciation from users seeking to restore energy, support their joints and bones, and improve overall resilience. With an average satisfaction rating of 4.5 out of 5 stars, this supplement continues to stand out for individuals looking to replenish their bodies with deeply nourishing, bioavailable nutrients.

Our review analysis reveals the most commonly reported benefits among users who shared a positive experience with beef bone and marrow. These reports highlight where users saw the most meaningful support. While results vary by individual, a higher percentage in the table below suggests a greater likelihood of experiencing that benefit, particularly if you have similar goals or concerns.

For instance, if 37% of reviewers mention improved energy, that suggests a strong user pattern of renewed stamina and reduced fatigue. These percentages are not guarantees but offer insight into where this supplement may be most impactful.

Below is a summary table of Beef Bone and Marrow's top benefits as reported by customers:

Benefit	%	Explanation
Energy Boost	37%	Users often report a noticeable increase in energy and endurance, with less fatigue throughout the day and improved stamina for daily activities.
Skin Health	24%	Many users describe better skin hydration, smoother texture, and a more radiant complexion, with some noting relief from dryness and skin fragility.
Joint Support	17%	A significant number of users experience greater flexibility, comfort, and ease of movement, particularly in knees, hips, and shoulders.
Bone Strength	12%	Some reviewers share that they feel greater skeletal support and resilience, especially during recovery or aging.
Cartilage Support	10%	Users mention added comfort in joints, attributing it to improved cartilage protection and cushioning during physical activity.

How to Use This Table

This table reflects the most common benefits experienced by users who reported positive results with beef bone and marrow. While everyone's experience will vary, the data can help you determine whether this supplement aligns with your needs.

If your goals include increasing energy, supporting your joints, or improving your skin, these figures suggest a strong track record in those areas. Many reviewers also mention compounding benefits when beef bone and marrow is taken consistently over time, especially when paired with other foundational nutrients like beef liver or collagen.

Think of this table as a guide, not a guarantee, to help you set realistic expectations and better understand what thousands of other users have experienced.

Beef Spleen

Grass-fed beef spleen is a rich, traditional food source that has long been valued for its role in supporting overall vitality. As one of the most concentrated natural sources of heme iron and vitamin B12, it provides essential building blocks for energy production and red blood cell formation. The spleen is also a key part of the immune system, and its nutrients help nourish the body's natural defenses.

Beef spleen supplements, derived from pasture-raised cattle, offer a highly bioavailable blend of iron, zinc, selenium, and other trace minerals that are often challenging to obtain in sufficient amounts through modern diets. These nutrients are critical for supporting oxygen transport, cellular repair, and immune readiness.

By incorporating beef spleen into a daily supplement routine, many individuals aim to enhance their energy, restore nutrient balance, and reinforce foundational health, particularly in areas related to blood and immune function. As with all organ-based nutrition, its benefits are best understood as part of a broader effort to nourish the body using whole-food, ancestral sources.

Science-Informed Beef Spleen Benefits

Supports Immune Function

The spleen is an essential organ in the lymphatic and immune systems, responsible for filtering the blood, managing immune cell populations, and removing old or damaged red blood cells. Nutritionally, beef spleen provides a concentrated source of key immune-supportive nutrients, including zinc and selenium. These minerals contribute to the maintenance of immune cell activity and help support the body's natural defense mechanisms.

Regular intake of beef spleen as part of a nutrient-diverse routine may help strengthen immune readiness by supplying the building blocks needed for white blood cell formation and proper immune modulation.

Promotes Healthy Iron and Red Blood Cell Levels

Beef spleen is one of the richest natural sources of heme iron, the form of iron most readily absorbed and utilized by the human body. Heme iron is critical for the formation of hemoglobin, the protein in red blood cells that transports oxygen throughout the body. In addition to iron, beef spleen also contains vitamin B12, which plays a vital role in red blood cell production and overall blood health.

By delivering these nutrients in their naturally occurring, food-based forms, beef spleen offers support for individuals seeking to maintain healthy iron levels and circulatory function. This may be particularly useful for those with dietary gaps or increased physiological demands.

Contributes to Sustained Energy and Vitality

Iron and vitamin B12 are fundamental to cellular energy metabolism. These nutrients help support mitochondrial activity, the process through which the body converts nutrients into usable energy. When nutritional intake of iron and B12 is inadequate, energy production can be impaired, contributing to feelings of fatigue or low stamina.

Beef spleen provides these nutrients in a bioavailable form, making it a practical option for individuals who wish to support energy levels through natural dietary strategies. Its nutrient profile may be especially relevant for those recovering from physical stress, long-term fatigue, or nutritional depletion.

Nutritional Support for Inflammatory Balance

Beef spleen naturally contains trace minerals such as zinc and selenium, which are involved in regulating the body's inflammatory processes. These nutrients play key roles in antioxidant defense systems and cellular repair mechanisms that help maintain a balanced response to physical stressors.

By offering nourishment that supports the body's own capacity for regulation and repair, beef spleen may assist those who are focused on maintaining a healthy inflammatory response as part of their wellness routine.

Provides Foundational Nutrients for Spleen and Lymphatic Support

From a nutritional perspective, consuming an organ such as spleen may provide proteins, enzymes, and cofactors that are uniquely suited to supporting the same organ system in the human body. While more research is needed to fully understand the implications, this traditional concept of "like supports like" remains an area of growing interest in holistic and ancestral health practices.

Beef spleen supplements deliver essential micronutrients and peptides that nourish the body's circulatory and immune pathways. This may offer targeted support for individuals seeking to maintain the health of the spleen and broader lymphatic function.

Customer-Reported Beef Spleen Benefits

Grass-fed beef spleen supplements have received enthusiastic feedback from individuals seeking to restore energy, improve iron levels, and support immune resilience. With a high overall rating of 4.6 out of 5 from thousands of verified users, this organ-based supplement has emerged as a natural option for people navigating fatigue, low iron status, and immune system imbalances.

Our in-depth analysis of customer experiences reveals a pattern of meaningful improvements, particularly in cases where traditional supplements or medications were poorly tolerated or ineffective. From those recovering from long-term nutrient depletion to individuals managing chronic conditions, beef spleen is often described as a turning point in their wellness journey. The data that follows highlights key patterns in how people are using this supplement, what they report feeling, and which benefits show up most consistently among positive reviews.

Use Case Patterns Observed

Many individuals turn to beef spleen supplements when dealing with persistent fatigue, low iron status, or reduced immune resilience. A significant number of users share that they had been struggling with low energy, frequent illness, or nutrient depletion, often after periods of intense stress, recovery, or dietary limitations.

Others began using beef spleen to support wellness during times of immune vulnerability, such as seasonal challenges or personal health transitions. Some mention long-standing issues with nutrient absorption or energy imbalance, which had left them searching for a gentle, food-based alternative to conventional iron pills.

It is also common for people to pair spleen with liver or bone marrow supplements when trying to support energy production, stamina, or general vitality. A few users describe giving it to loved ones who needed additional strength during demanding life circumstances, seeing it as a whole-food way to nourish the body deeply.

Feedback Insights

The emotional tone across positive reviews is one of deep relief and renewed hope. Many users describe beef spleen as "life-changing" or say it brought them back from a state of depletion they once believed was permanent. A number of reviewers share that their energy returned after years of struggle, saying things like "I finally feel like a human being again" or "my energy came back and I didn't need to nap just to get through the day."

Improvements in iron levels are often noted in test results, with several users documenting measurable increases in hemoglobin and ferritin. These changes are not just numerical. People mention visible shifts, like color returning to their skin, their hands warming up, and their cheeks gaining a healthy flush. Others talk about hair regrowth, saying they were brought to tears after seeing hair come back for the first time in years.

Many also express gratitude that this supplement did not cause the stomach upset they experienced with traditional iron pills. One reviewer summed it up by saying, "This is how nature intended your body to get nutrients, through real food." Others commented on the noticeable boost to immune resilience, especially when surrounded by illness. For some, it helped them avoid frequent infections or recover more quickly than expected.

Emotional language is strong across many reviews. Words like "grateful," "thankful," "in tears," "miracle," and "hope restored" appear again and again. This supplement is often described not just as effective, but as a turning point that gave people their vitality and confidence back.

Most Reported Benefits from Review Analysis

Beef spleen is often selected by those looking to support iron levels, boost energy, and reinforce immune resilience. With an overall satisfaction rating of **4.6 out of 5 stars**, this nutrient-rich supplement continues to resonate with users who seek whole-food sources of strength and vitality.

We analyzed thousands of positive reviews to identify which benefits were most frequently mentioned by satisfied customers. The percentages below reflect how often each benefit came up in user feedback. A higher percentage may suggest a greater likelihood of noticing that result, especially if your needs are similar to those of the reviewers.

For example, if 30% of positive reviewers highlighted iron support, this indicates a strong trend among users who felt improvements in energy, endurance, or nutrient balance after adding beef spleen to their routine.

Below is a summary table of Beef Spleen's top benefits as reported by customers:

Benefit	%	Explanation
Iron Support	30%	Many reviewers noted improvements in iron-related metrics, including better stamina, less lightheadedness, and a renewed sense of physical vitality.

Benefit	%	Explanation
Energy Boost	27%	Users frequently described a meaningful lift in daily energy, reduced fatigue, and a return of motivation or mental clarity.
Blood Health	23%	Numerous individuals shared that they felt stronger, more balanced, and more resilient, attributing these shifts to perceived improvements in circulation and nutrient delivery.
Low Iron Recovery	10%	A portion of reviewers mentioned experiences of feeling more robust and stable, particularly after seeking natural alternatives for restoring iron status.
Immune Resilience	10%	Users reported feeling better equipped to navigate seasonal or environmental challenges, with some noting fewer setbacks and quicker recovery times.

How to Use This Table

The figures shown here reflect patterns from those who shared positive experiences with beef spleen supplements. While individual results may vary, this data helps illustrate where users most often see benefits.

If your personal goals include supporting energy, blood-building nutrients, or foundational immune strength, these insights may help guide your expectations. As always, results can depend on consistency, lifestyle, and how the supplement fits into your broader wellness approach.

This summary is not intended as medical advice, but rather as a reflection of real-world user feedback gathered from verified reviews. Always speak with a healthcare provider before starting any new supplement routine.

Beef Lung

Beef lung supplements offer a nutrient-rich way to support respiratory function, oxygen use, and general vitality. Traditionally, lung tissue from pasture-raised animals was included in ancestral diets to provide nourishment for individuals engaged in strenuous activity or living in high-demand environments. Today, beef lung remains valued for its role in offering targeted nutritional support for lung health and energy metabolism.

Derived from grass-fed cattle, these supplements are a natural source of proteins, peptides, and bioavailable co-factors that play important roles in oxygen delivery and cellular resilience. Many people incorporate beef lung into their routines as part of a broader effort to maintain healthy respiratory function and support physical stamina.

Rather than relying on processed or synthetic ingredients, beef lung provides a whole-food approach rooted in traditional wisdom. For those seeking to align modern wellness goals with time-honored nutritional practices, it offers a convenient and meaningful addition to a nutrient-focused lifestyle.

Science-Informed Beef Lung Benefits

Nutritional Support for Respiratory Function and Lung Structure

Beef lung is a concentrated source of peptides, proteins, and naturally occurring co-factors that contribute to the maintenance of healthy lung tissue. These nutrients help support the structural components of the lungs and may assist in preserving normal respiratory function. Historically, traditional diets included lung tissue as a way to nourish this vital organ system, especially in environments that placed greater physical or environmental stress on the lungs.

Helps Facilitate Efficient Oxygen Transport and Physical Endurance

The lungs are essential for oxygen exchange, supplying oxygen to the bloodstream so that it can be used for energy production throughout the body. Nutrients found in beef lung help support the body's ability to maintain efficient oxygen delivery, which is especially important during periods of physical activity or recovery. Individuals seeking to improve stamina or reduce feelings of fatigue often turn to lung-rich organ supplements as part of their wellness strategy to enhance oxygen availability.

Supports the Body's Natural Immune Barriers

The respiratory system plays a central role in the body's first line of defense. Nutrients within beef lung, including tissue-specific peptides and immune-supporting proteins, may help reinforce the natural barriers that protect the lungs. While these nutrients are not intended to prevent or treat illness, they contribute to a well-nourished internal environment that supports the immune system's normal function.

Helps Maintain a Balanced Inflammatory Response in the Lungs

Beef lung provides bioavailable compounds that are believed to support a balanced immune and inflammatory response. Maintaining this balance is important for lung comfort, especially for those regularly exposed to airborne irritants or environmental stressors.

While not intended to treat any specific respiratory condition, this nutritional support may complement efforts to keep the lungs functioning optimally.

Provides Nutrients That May Aid in Recovery Support

Recovering from stressors that impact the respiratory system requires adequate nutritional support. The peptides and proteins found in beef lung offer building blocks that may help support the body's natural repair processes. This can be especially valuable for individuals focused on rebuilding strength and resilience following periods of respiratory strain.

Customer-Reported Beef Lung Benefits

Beef lung supplements have earned high praise from thousands of users who report noticeable improvements in their breathing, energy, and overall wellness. With a strong average satisfaction rating of 4.7 out of 5 stars, users frequently highlight how these capsules helped them breathe more freely, recover from respiratory challenges, and restore a sense of vitality. While individual responses vary, many people find that consistent use leads to clearer lungs, deeper sleep, improved stamina, and a greater ability to engage in daily life without discomfort or shortness of breath.

Our analysis of verified 4- and 5-star reviews reveals the most frequently reported benefits from those who experienced positive results. These percentages represent how often each benefit was mentioned in successful outcomes, offering a helpful window into the kinds of improvements users may experience.

Use Case Patterns Observed

Beef lung supplements are often chosen by individuals dealing with respiratory concerns, such as lingering coughs, shortness of breath, reduced lung function, or environmental irritants. Many users mention taking beef lung as part of their recovery after respiratory illnesses, extended fatigue, or long-term breathing issues. Some specifically turn to it following seasonal changes, wildfire smoke, past infections, or chronic conditions that left their lungs feeling weak or constricted.

Several people begin using beef lung as a preventive measure to maintain healthy respiratory function, especially those in physically demanding jobs or living in areas with poor air quality. Others incorporate it into wellness protocols for improving energy, oxygen circulation, and general vitality, often in combination with other organ supplements.

Feedback Insights

Customers consistently express deep relief and gratitude for the improvements they've felt. One recurring theme is the emotional transformation that accompanies easier breathing. Users describe the experience as "freeing," "incredible," and even "life-changing." Many are surprised by how quickly they feel a difference, sometimes within days, noting deeper breaths, less coughing, clearer airways, and better oxygen flow. Words like "finally," "hopeful," and "I can breathe again" appear frequently, reflecting the emotional weight of long-term respiratory struggles.

Several users describe a return to daily activities they previously avoided, such as walking, climbing stairs, or playing with their children. Improved sleep, reduced reliance on inhalers, and fewer flare-ups from allergies or past infections were also noted with enthusiasm. For those who had nearly given up on finding relief, the supplement offered renewed optimism and a sense that they were finally on the right path.

Most Reported Benefits from Review Analysis

To better understand what users are actually experiencing, we conducted a deep analysis of verified customer reviews, focusing on the benefits most frequently mentioned by satisfied users. The table below reflects the distribution of reported benefits across thousands of positive experiences. While individual results will always vary, a higher percentage suggests a more consistent pattern of benefit shared by others.

For example, 29% of reviewers specifically mentioned improvements in lung health and breathing capacity, suggesting that if respiratory support is your goal, beef lung may be especially worth considering. In addition, many users noted increases in daily energy and a greater sense of ease during physical activity, pointing to a broader role in enhancing endurance and oxygen use.

Below is a summary table of beef lung's top benefits as reported by customers:

Benefit	%	Explanation
Lung health	29%	Many users report improved lung function, better breathing, and stronger respiratory health.
Energy boost	26%	Increased stamina and vitality, with users feeling more active and less fatigued.
Breathing support	21%	Enhanced breathing capacity, making physical activities easier and more comfortable.

Benefit	%	Explanation
Respiratory Comfort	14%	Users with asthma and respiratory conditions report noticeable improvements in symptoms.
Immune support	10%	Strengthened immune function, with users experiencing fewer illnesses and faster recovery.

How to Use This Guide

If you're exploring beef lung to support respiratory wellness, boost energy, or enhance daily breathing, these real-world insights offer a helpful starting point. The percentages above reflect how often each benefit was mentioned by users who shared a positive experience. While not a promise of results, they do highlight the most common areas where people have found value.

It's also worth noting that many users report experiencing multiple benefits at once. For some, the positive effects appeared within a few days; for others, consistent use over several weeks brought gradual but meaningful change. Whether you're recovering from respiratory challenges, seeking better stamina, or simply looking for ways to support lung health naturally, beef lung stands out as a well-regarded option among those on a similar path.

Beef Adrenal

Grass-fed beef adrenal supplements offer a whole-food source of nutrients traditionally valued for supporting the body's natural stress response, energy production, and hormonal equilibrium. The adrenal glands are small but vital structures that help regulate key processes such as fluid balance, metabolism, and the body's ability to adapt to physical or emotional stress.

Sourced from pasture-raised cattle, beef adrenal provides naturally occurring bioactive compounds, including peptides and co-factors, that are uniquely concentrated in adrenal tissue. These nutrients are believed to help nourish adrenal function and promote a greater sense of resilience during times of fatigue, tension, or heightened demands.

Many people include beef adrenal supplements as part of their wellness routine when looking to maintain steady energy, support a healthy stress response, or encourage internal balance in a holistic way. For those navigating demanding lifestyles or seeking a more traditional approach to restoring vitality, beef adrenal offers targeted support from one of the body's core regulatory systems.

Science-Informed Beef Adrenal Benefits

Supports the Body's Natural Stress Response

The adrenal glands are responsible for producing key hormones such as cortisol and adrenaline, which play an essential role in how the body adapts to physical, emotional, and environmental stress. These hormones influence energy regulation, mood stability, metabolic function, and immune coordination. Beef adrenal supplements contain naturally occurring peptides and nutrients sourced from whole adrenal tissue, offering direct nutritional support to this critical system.

By nourishing the adrenal glands with tissue-specific compounds, this supplement may help the body better adapt to everyday stressors. Individuals with demanding schedules or high stress levels often turn to adrenal-based supplements to support a more balanced stress response and promote a sense of inner steadiness during times of challenge.

Promotes Sustained Energy and Vitality

Fatigue and low energy can be signs of systemic strain, especially when stress becomes chronic. The adrenal glands are involved in sustaining daily energy by regulating the balance of cortisol and related compounds. Beef adrenal supplements offer a source of nutrients such as vitamin B12, zinc, and co-factors that contribute to cellular energy metabolism. These nutrients are essential for converting food into usable energy and may reduce the overall burden on adrenal function during periods of high demand.

People seeking to maintain stamina throughout the day, whether due to lifestyle pressure or low vitality, often incorporate adrenal tissue into their wellness routines as part of a broader strategy for promoting steady, sustainable energy.

Helps Maintain Hormonal Balance

Beyond stress hormones, the adrenal glands also produce aldosterone and other compounds that influence blood pressure, metabolism, and fluid balance. Beef adrenal supplements provide naturally occurring proteins, amino acids, and minerals that serve as foundational building blocks for hormone production and regulation.

Supporting adrenal gland nutrition may contribute to a more stable internal environment, which is especially useful for individuals navigating periods of hormonal fluctuation or seeking to optimize endocrine system function from a food-based perspective.

Nutritional Support for Immune Health

Prolonged stress and adrenal strain are often associated with reduced immune efficiency. The adrenal glands interact with immune-regulating systems through the release of glucocorticoids and other compounds that modulate inflammation and immune signaling. Beef adrenal supplements offer tissue-specific nutrients that can help support the body's natural immune readiness, especially during times of recovery or elevated stress.

By providing nutrients that indirectly nourish immune coordination, beef adrenal may be a valuable tool in a comprehensive wellness plan for individuals aiming to feel more resilient and supported.

Contributes to Electrolyte and Fluid Balance

One of the lesser-known functions of the adrenal glands is the regulation of electrolytes, particularly sodium and potassium, through the hormone aldosterone. These minerals are essential for proper hydration, nerve transmission, muscle function, and cardiovascular rhythm. When adrenal function is compromised, electrolyte balance can be affected, leading to symptoms such as salt cravings, lightheadedness, or dehydration.

Beef adrenal supplements offer nutritional support that may help maintain optimal adrenal output and fluid regulation, making them a thoughtful option for those looking to promote metabolic balance, hydration, and physical performance.

Customer-Reported Beef Adrenal Benefits

Beef adrenal supplements have quickly earned a passionate following among those seeking more sustainable energy, emotional balance, and recovery from the wear and tear of modern stress. With an average user rating of 4.8 out of 5 and thousands of enthusiastic reviews, it's clear that beef adrenal has become a trusted tool in many wellness journeys. Unlike quick fixes or stimulants, this supplement is consistently described as offering steady, grounding support that helps people feel more capable, calm, and clear throughout the day. Whether dealing with lingering fatigue, stress-related burnout, or hormonal imbalance, many users report feeling more like themselves again, sometimes for the first time in years.

Use Case Patterns Observed

Many individuals begin using beef adrenal during times of chronic fatigue, emotional exhaustion, or intense life stress. Several reviewers shared that they were navigating burnout, adrenal fatigue, or low morning energy and were searching for something to help restore resilience. Others were recovering from long-term stress, post-viral fatigue, or hormonal shifts and found that beef adrenal helped them feel more balanced and alert. The supplement is often used in the morning to support all-day energy or alongside thyroid and liver support for a more complete approach to hormonal and metabolic wellness. A notable pattern is the shift from reactive solutions, like caffeine or synthetic adrenal formulas, to whole-food support that users say feels more natural and lasting.

Feedback Insights

Emotional language runs deep in these reviews. Many describe a sense of "finally feeling calm again," "getting their life back," or "waking up with purpose." One user wrote that after years of feeling wired but tired, this was the first supplement that helped them relax and energize at the same time. Others speak of clearer thinking, more stable moods, and a noticeable return of motivation, what one reviewer called "a steady energy that doesn't crash."

Another common theme is emotional relief. Some users shared that their nervous system felt calmer, their mood more grounded, and their ability to respond to daily stress had improved significantly. One reviewer described tears of gratitude, finally feeling peace in their body after months of feeling like they were in constant survival mode. Others described less brain fog, better focus, and being able to sleep more deeply and wake up feeling rested.

For those managing hormonal issues, adrenal support is often paired with thyroid and liver supplements. Users consistently report that the combination helped improve their results, emotional balance, and overall physical stamina. Many also mentioned that once they addressed adrenal health, other parts of their wellness plan began to fall into place more easily.

Overall, beef adrenal is not seen as a stimulant or a quick solution, but as a gentle, powerful source of nourishment for a body that has been running on empty. And in a fast-paced world where burnout is increasingly common, that kind of support feels more valuable than ever.

Most Reported Benefits from Review Analysis

To better understand how beef adrenal is being used in real life, we conducted a detailed analysis of verified customer reviews, focusing on the benefits most frequently mentioned by users who reported positive outcomes. The table below reflects the distribution of those benefits across thousands of experiences. While individual responses vary, a higher percentage suggests a more consistent trend across different users.

For instance, 43% of reviewers specifically mentioned improvements related to adrenal function, such as increased stamina, improved stress response, or greater day-to-day resilience. Energy support, stress regulation, and sleep quality were also consistently highlighted, suggesting that beef adrenal may play a valuable role in helping people restore balance and feel more grounded during periods of physical or emotional depletion.

Below is a summary table of Beef Adrenal's top benefits as reported by customers:

Benefit	%	Explanation
Adrenal Support	43%	Users often report feeling more balanced and resilient, with noticeable support for adrenal function and recovery from chronic stress.
Energy Boost	27%	Many experience a steady, sustained increase in energy throughout the day, without the highs and lows associated with caffeine or stimulants.
Stress Resilience	12%	Several users describe an improved ability to cope with daily challenges, with a greater sense of calm and less overwhelm.
Sleep Improvement	10%	Some reviewers noted deeper, more restful sleep and improved recovery, particularly when taken in the morning to regulate stress patterns.
Fatigue Reduction	8%	Users with long-term tiredness or burnout say they feel more recharged and capable of handling demanding days with greater ease.

How to Use This Guide

If you're considering beef adrenal to support energy, stress management, or hormonal balance, these insights can help guide your expectations. The percentages listed reflect how frequently each benefit was mentioned by satisfied users. While not a guarantee of individual outcomes, they offer a real-world snapshot of what others have commonly experienced.

Many users report feeling multiple benefits at once, often noticing subtle improvements in energy, focus, mood, and recovery after a few days to several weeks of consistent use. For those navigating high levels of stress or seeking to replenish after burnout, beef adrenal is often described as a natural, steady source of strength, offering support that builds gently over time rather than delivering a quick fix.

Beef Testicles

Grass-fed beef testicle supplements provide a concentrated source of bioavailable nutrients traditionally associated with male reproductive and hormonal health. Long used in various cultures as part of ancestral diets to support vitality, strength, and reproductive function, beef testicles contain naturally occurring peptides, enzymes, and co-factors that help nourish the body's endocrine system.

Sourced from pasture-raised cattle, these supplements offer a convenient way to incorporate this nutrient-dense organ into a modern wellness routine. They are often chosen by individuals looking to support physical performance, maintain healthy hormone levels, or promote overall male vitality through a food-based, natural approach.

Science-Informed Beef Testicles Benefits

Supports Testosterone Production Naturally

Beef testicle supplements contain naturally occurring nutrients that may support the body's ability to produce testosterone, including cholesterol, zinc, and specific peptides. These compounds play an essential role in hormone synthesis and are particularly important for maintaining healthy testosterone levels in men.

Many individuals turn to beef testicle supplements as part of a holistic approach to support their energy, strength, and mood, particularly as they age or during times when hormonal support is needed.

Promotes Reproductive Health and Sperm Quality

Beef testicles offer a rich source of nutrients such as selenium, zinc, and amino acids that are known to contribute to sperm health. These nutrients have been associated with healthy sperm motility, structure, and count, all of which are important factors in male reproductive function.

For those looking to nourish the reproductive system through food-based support, beef testicle supplements provide a nutrient-dense option grounded in traditional dietary practices.

Supports Muscle Health and Physical Performance

Testosterone plays a key role in muscle maintenance, energy metabolism, and physical endurance. By providing nutritional components that may support testosterone balance, beef testicle supplements are often used by individuals who engage in strength training, athletic activity, or physically demanding routines.

This nutritional support may contribute to better workout performance, enhanced recovery, and greater resilience to physical stressors.

Contributes to Sexual Well-Being

Many users associate beef testicle supplements with enhanced vitality and sexual confidence. This may be due to the role testosterone plays in regulating libido, performance, and overall sexual function.

By offering nutritional support for hormone regulation, beef testicle supplements can help support the foundational systems that influence sexual wellness.

Nutritional Support for Endocrine Balance

Beef testicles are naturally rich in vitamins and minerals that help support overall hormonal balance, including vitamin B12, selenium, and zinc. These nutrients are involved in the function of the endocrine system, which regulates mood, energy levels, and metabolic processes.

Regular use of beef testicle supplements may support mental clarity, balanced energy throughout the day, and a general sense of well-being, especially when used alongside other nutrient-rich whole food supplements.

Customer-Reported Beef Testicles Benefits

Beef testicle supplements have become a trusted addition to many men's wellness routines, particularly among those seeking to support vitality, stamina, and hormonal health through food-based supplementation. With an impressive average rating of 4.5 out of 5, these supplements are consistently praised for helping users feel more energized, focused, and confident in their daily lives. Many men describe noticeable shifts in how they perform physically and mentally, often reporting that they feel more like themselves again. For those dealing with the effects of age-related hormone decline, high stress, or demanding physical routines, beef testicle supplements offer a natural way to feel stronger and more resilient.

Use Case Patterns Observed

Beef testicle supplements are most often used by men navigating changes in energy, motivation, or physical performance, especially in midlife or after periods of chronic stress. Some discover the solution after years of experimenting with other testosterone support options, reporting that this supplement provided the missing link. Others turn to it while recovering from hormonal imbalances or seeking to rebuild strength after burnout or illness.

A consistent theme is the desire to restore baseline vitality. Reviewers often mention pairing these supplements with improved diet, strength training, or functional testing. In several cases, men who had undergone testosterone checking noted significant changes after consistent use. This makes beef testicle supplements especially appealing to those who value measurable progress and are working toward long-term hormonal balance and performance optimization.

Feedback Insights

Across thousands of reviews, users describe their experiences using vivid and emotionally resonant language. The most common feeling expressed is one of renewed energy and motivation. Many reviewers say they feel "better than they have in years" and that they now get through the day with greater stamina, sharper focus, and fewer crashes. One user put it simply: "I feel like I've gotten myself back."

Another powerful theme is confidence and restoration of identity. For men who felt their drive, strength, or sense of masculinity had faded, this supplement was often credited with helping them reconnect with their physical and emotional power. One reviewer shared that his "productivity has majorly increased" and another said, "I didn't realize how much this was missing until it was back."

Sexual wellness is also frequently highlighted. Men report feeling more present, responsive, and confident in intimate settings. In many cases, this was described as part of a broader improvement in hormonal balance and vitality rather than as an isolated effect. Several reviewers mentioned positive changes confirmed by lab tests, including increased testosterone levels and improved overall wellness markers.

What sets this solution apart for many users is not just the outcome, but the emotional relief of finding something that finally works. Some reviewers, including those recovering from stress-related health issues or hormone therapy, expressed gratitude and even surprise at how meaningful the changes were. In the words of one longtime user: "From feeling like I was dying to feeling amazing, it's just miraculous."

Whether taken alone or as part of a full organ supplement protocol, beef testicle supplements stand out as a deeply supportive and empowering option for men seeking natural strength and balance.

Most Reported Benefits from Review Analysis

To better understand how users are responding to beef testicle supplements in real-world use, we analyzed thousands of verified reviews to identify the most frequently mentioned benefits among satisfied users. The table below highlights the distribution of these benefits based on positive experiences. While everyone's body responds differently, a higher percentage reflects a more consistent pattern of support that many users have shared.

For example, 56% of users highlighted noticeable improvements in energy and stamina, suggesting that if you are seeking greater physical vitality or reduced fatigue, this supplement may be especially helpful. Likewise, support for muscle development and strength was mentioned regularly, reflecting its appeal to those focused on performance, recovery, and longevity.

Below is a summary table of Beef Testicles' top benefits as reported by customers:

Benefit	%	Explanation
Energy boost	56%	Many users report a significant increase in energy and stamina, reducing sluggishness and improving overall vitality.
Energy Boost	56%	Users frequently report a significant and sustained lift in daily energy, improved stamina, and reduced dependence on caffeine or stimulants.
Muscle Support	19%	Many reviewers mention better workout recovery, enhanced endurance, and increased lean muscle development.
Testosterone Support	9%	Some users observe noticeable changes in testosterone-related markers, including motivation, libido, and hormone test results.
Strength Increase	9%	Users often describe feeling physically stronger, with improved gym performance and resilience in daily activities.

How to Use This Guide

If you are considering beef testicle supplements for specific goals such as boosting energy, supporting testosterone, or enhancing performance, the insights above offer a useful starting point. These percentages reflect how often users mentioned each benefit after a positive experience, not a guaranteed outcome. However, they do highlight the areas where this supplement has earned the most consistent praise.

Many users also report experiencing multiple benefits at once, especially when taken consistently over several weeks. Energy, strength, and hormonal support often go hand in hand, and reviewers frequently note that results build gradually and steadily. Whether you are looking to restore physical vitality, sharpen your focus, or support your body's natural balance, beef testicle supplements may offer meaningful support grounded in real user experience and traditional nutritional wisdom.

Beef Uterus and Ovaries

Grass-fed beef uterus and ovary supplements offer a concentrated source of bioavailable nutrients traditionally associated with supporting female reproductive function and hormonal health. In many ancestral dietary practices, these organs were consumed to help nourish the body during times of reproductive transition, from menstruation to menopause.

Sourced from pasture-raised cattle, these supplements contain naturally occurring peptides, proteins, and cofactors that may help the body maintain hormonal balance and overall reproductive wellness. Many women seeking to support their natural rhythm, promote cycle regularity, or maintain vitality during life's hormonal shifts have found these whole-food supplements to be a valuable part of their broader wellness routine.

Science-Informed Beef Uterus and Ovaries Benefits

Supports Hormonal Health and Balance

Beef uterus and ovary supplements contain naturally occurring peptides, proteins, and micronutrients that play a role in supporting the endocrine system. Nutrients such as vitamin B12, zinc, and selenium are known to contribute to normal hormonal activity and energy metabolism. When included as part of a nutrient-rich wellness routine, these organ supplements may help the body maintain hormonal equilibrium during times of change or stress.

This type of support may be especially useful for individuals navigating transitions such as menopause or seeking nutritional strategies to maintain overall reproductive wellness.

Nutritional Support for Fertility and Reproductive Function

The ovary and uterus are both rich in structural proteins and cofactors that, when consumed in whole-food form, provide a wide spectrum of nutrients specific to female reproductive physiology. These include bioavailable amino acids, trace minerals like selenium and zinc, and naturally occurring enzymes that may help nourish tissues and support cellular integrity.

This broad nutritional profile can offer targeted support for those looking to maintain a healthy reproductive system and optimize preconception wellness through diet and lifestyle.

Helps Maintain Comfort During Menopause

The transition through menopause involves a gradual decline in hormone production, which may influence energy, mood, and physical comfort. While beef ovary and uterus supplements do not contain hormones in therapeutic quantities, they do offer essential nutrients that help the body maintain its natural processes during this phase.

By supplying supportive building blocks for tissue repair, metabolic balance, and resilience, these supplements may contribute to a more balanced sense of well-being in midlife and beyond.

Promotes Cycle Regularity Through Nutrient Density

For individuals experiencing irregular or inconsistent menstrual cycles, nutrient intake can be a key factor. Beef uterus and ovary supplements deliver bioavailable compounds involved in hormone regulation, including vitamin B12, iron, and collagen. These nutrients support cellular health, blood production, and connective tissue repair, all of which are important for cycle regulation.

While not a replacement for medical treatment, these supplements can be a complementary nutritional tool in supporting menstrual health as part of a balanced routine.

Supports Tissue Health in Reproductive Organs

The uterus and ovaries contain dense connective tissues and specialized proteins that, when consumed, provide organ-specific nourishment. Collagen, elastin, and bioactive peptides from these tissues may support structural integrity and resilience in the body's own reproductive organs.

This form of whole-food nutrition is particularly relevant for individuals recovering from childbirth, supporting postnatal wellness, or seeking to maintain the integrity of reproductive tissues over time.

Customer-Reported Uterus and Ovary Benefits

Beef uterus and ovary supplements have earned a strong reputation among women seeking natural support for hormonal balance, cycle regularity, and reproductive vitality. With an impressive customer rating of 4.5 out of 5, these supplements are praised not only for their quality but also for the meaningful changes users report in their energy, mood, menstrual comfort, and sense of well-being. While individual experiences vary, the feedback paints a clear picture of renewed confidence and restored inner balance. Many women describe the experience as "feeling like myself again" or finally finding something that truly makes a difference after trying other approaches.

This supplement is not framed as a miracle fix, but as a steady and effective source of nourishment for women at various stages of life, from those navigating perimenopause to others managing the effects of hormonal fluctuations, medication changes, or long-standing imbalance. For some, it became the turning point after months or even years of frustration. The changes often emerge gradually, but with deep impact: more stable mood, healthier cycles, improved sleep, and even subtle shifts in skin, weight, and vitality that help women reconnect with their bodies in a positive way.

Use Case Patterns Observed

Women often turn to beef uterus and ovary supplements when facing symptoms tied to hormonal shifts or reproductive discomfort. For some, it starts after experiencing irregular cycles, heavy cramping, or missing periods altogether. Others discover it during perimenopause or after medical interventions, which may have impacted their natural hormonal rhythm. A number of users were already working with naturopaths or taking other supplements but hadn't seen meaningful change until adding this product.

Several reviewers describe it as a last attempt after years of fatigue, brain fog, mood swings, or unexplainable weight plateaus. Others were simply curious about natural, nutrient-dense support for menstrual health, libido, and vitality. Some shared that they began taking it for specific issues like dryness, bloating, or emotional sensitivity and were surprised by how many areas of health improved at once. Whether taken as part of a broader wellness protocol or on its own, this supplement is often described as life-enhancing, even at lower doses.

Feedback Insights

Reviewers frequently express gratitude and even amazement at how much better they feel after using beef uterus and ovary supplements. One woman said she had not had a period in 19 months, yet after one month on this supplement, she experienced what she described as the most comfortable, balanced cycle of her life, with no cramping, no heaviness, and a sense of hormonal ease she hadn't felt in years. Others mention powerful emotional improvements, including phrases like "I feel like me again," "my essence is back," and "I finally feel well."

A common theme is improved energy, often described as "amazing," "noticeable within days," or "like a reset." Sleep is another area where women report meaningful change, waking up more rested and refreshed. Several note smoother, less painful periods, fewer mood swings, and even improved skin tone. One user mentioned that after switching to a different brand, her energy declined, reinforcing how strongly she felt about returning to this one.

Reviewers also reflect on the emotional and personal impact of these changes. They describe feeling calmer, more emotionally stable, and more connected to their partners. A few even joked about unexpected tears or mood surges from hormonal shifts, not in a negative way, but as evidence that the supplements were working on a deep level. For many, the supplement brought more than just symptom relief; it brought a sense of restoration and empowerment.

One woman summed it up simply: "I will never not take this."

Most Reported Benefits from Review Analysis

To better understand how this supplement supports real users, we analyzed thousands of verified reviews to identify the benefits most frequently mentioned by satisfied customers. The table below reflects the distribution of commonly reported outcomes across positive experiences. While each individual may respond differently, a higher percentage indicates a more consistent pattern reported by others.

For instance, 60% of reviewers shared that they experienced a noticeable increase in energy and vitality. Many described this shift as one of the first signs that their body was responding well to the supplement. Others noted more emotional steadiness and smoother monthly rhythms, suggesting a broad sense of support across different wellness needs.

Below is a summary table of the most reported benefits of Beef Uterus and Ovary Supplements:

Benefit	%	Explanation
Energy Boost	60%	Users often report feeling more energized and less drained, with renewed motivation and improved daily stamina.
Mood Balance	15%	Many share feeling more emotionally stable, with fewer mood fluctuations and a greater sense of calm.
Monthly Cycle Support	9%	Users note that their cycles feel more predictable, easier to manage, and sometimes more comfortable overall.
Hormonal Harmony	9%	Customers describe improvements in how their body feels overall, attributing it to better hormonal alignment.
General Reproductive Support	8%	Reviewers frequently mention feeling more connected to their body's natural rhythm and noticing positive shifts in well-being.

How to Use This Guide

If you are considering this supplement to support energy, mood, or hormonal health, this analysis can serve as a helpful starting point. These figures do not guarantee specific results but offer insight into which areas of wellness users most often report experiencing benefits.

It is also common for users to report more than one benefit at a time. Many found that the effects became more noticeable with consistent use over several weeks. Whether your goals include supporting energy levels, maintaining balance, or enhancing overall vitality, this supplement has become a valued addition to many women's self-care routines.

Beef Thymus

Beef thymus supplements, sourced from grass-fed, pasture-raised cattle, offer a concentrated source of bioavailable nutrients traditionally valued for their role in supporting immune resilience and vitality. In many ancestral cultures, the thymus was considered an important part of a nose-to-tail approach to wellness, valued for its nutritional density and alignment with the principle of "like supports like."

The thymus plays a key role during early life in the development of the body's immune system, particularly in the maturation of certain white blood cells. Although this organ becomes less active over time, it remains symbolically and nutritionally linked to the body's natural defense systems.

Beef thymus supplements provide peptides, proteins, and micronutrients that may complement a wellness routine aimed at supporting balance, energy, and immune system integrity. Many people choose thymus as part of a broader strategy to promote whole-body wellness and to nourish systems that help maintain long-term resilience.

Science-Informed Beef Thymus Benefits

Supports Natural Immune Function

The thymus plays a central role in the body's early immune development by contributing to the maturation of T-cells, a type of white blood cell involved in recognizing and responding to external challenges. While the thymus becomes less active over time, its foundational influence on immune system function remains significant. Beef thymus supplements contain naturally occurring peptides, cofactors, and micronutrients that are thought to support the body's natural immune processes. These nutrients may help maintain immune vigilance, especially during times when the body needs added resilience.

Promotes Immune System Balance

Nutritional support from glandular supplements like beef thymus may help promote immune system balance. Rather than simply stimulating or suppressing immune activity, the unique compounds found in thymus tissue are believed to help modulate responses in a way that supports overall immune integrity. This type of support can be beneficial for individuals seeking to maintain equilibrium in their immune function during seasonal changes, lifestyle stress, or shifts in their wellness routine.

Helps Support Post-Stress and Post-Illness Recovery

Periods of high stress or extended health challenges may leave the body feeling depleted or sluggish. The thymus has been traditionally associated with recovery and rebuilding during such times. Nutrients and peptides found in beef thymus may provide foundational support as part of a nutritional strategy to help the body regain vitality, support energy levels, and promote a sense of restored well-being after fatigue or strain.

Contributes to a Calmer Immune Response

Many people are concerned about how their immune system reacts to everyday triggers such as environmental irritants or dietary stressors. Beef thymus supplements may provide gentle nutritional support that helps the body respond with greater ease. Some peptides found in thymus tissue have been studied for their role in maintaining a balanced inflammatory response, which can be important for comfort and tolerance when the body faces occasional internal or external stressors.

Nourishes the Immune-Endocrine Connection

The thymus is part of a complex network of glands that includes the adrenals and other components of the endocrine system. This network influences how the body responds to physical and emotional stress. By providing essential cofactors, glandular supplements such as beef thymus may help nourish this broader system, offering support for those aiming to maintain clarity, energy, and equilibrium in demanding times. This kind of nutritional support may be particularly useful for individuals who prioritize endocrine-immune harmony as part of their wellness goals.

Customer-Reported Beef Thymus Benefits

Beef thymus supplements are earning strong praise from those seeking support for immune balance, energy recovery, and relief from chronic sensitivities. With an average satisfaction rating of 4.6 out of 5, these supplements have become a trusted part of wellness routines for people navigating complex immune responses, persistent fatigue, and histamine sensitivity. Many users describe feeling surprised, sometimes even amazed, by how quickly their bodies responded, especially when other approaches had fallen short.

Through the lens of thousands of positive reviews, one thing becomes clear: this is not just another immune support supplement. Customers are turning to beef thymus during times of immune exhaustion, seasonal challenges, and after long periods of not feeling like themselves. The feedback is often emotional and deeply personal, reflecting a profound sense of relief and renewed vitality that some describe as life-changing.

Use Case Patterns Observed

Many customers begin using beef thymus after struggling with ongoing immune challenges, including sensitivity to environmental triggers, recurrent seasonal discomfort, or a general sense of immune imbalance. A large portion of users report turning to this supplement after exhausting other options, often in search of natural alternatives that feel more in tune with their body's rhythms.

Several reviews come from individuals recovering from significant immune stress or fatigue. This includes people navigating complex or chronic wellness concerns, as well as those experiencing energy crashes, brain fog, or prolonged recovery periods. For these users, thymus is seen as a tool for restoring resilience, particularly when used alongside other foundational organ supplements.

Another major group includes people exploring support for histamine-related symptoms or inflammatory responses. These users often report noticeable changes in allergy severity, skin comfort, or sinus congestion. In some cases, customers also describe benefits for mood, mental clarity, and overall daily energy, suggesting a broad systemic effect that extends beyond the immune system alone.

Feedback Insights

The emotional tone of the feedback is both enthusiastic and deeply grateful. Many users describe feeling "like themselves again" or "back to living" after long periods of discomfort. Words like "hopeful," "euphoric," and "grateful beyond words" appear repeatedly, underscoring the depth of transformation experienced by some.

Several users report surprise at how quickly their bodies responded, sometimes noticing changes in sinus pressure, fatigue, or mental clarity within hours or days. Others describe more gradual shifts that unfold over weeks, such as deeper sleep, less congestion, reduced inflammation, or calmer skin. Even those managing long-standing immune or histamine-related issues express optimism, sharing stories of steady improvement and reduced need for antihistamines or over-the-counter medications.

Parents mention improvements in their children's energy, sleep, or tolerance to allergens, while older adults describe feeling more alert, steady, and energetic. For those who had tried many different supplements without success, the response to beef thymus often feels like a breakthrough. Some even credit it with restoring hope after years of trial and error.

What unites these stories is the sense of regaining control, of finally finding something that supports their body in a way that feels natural, effective, and sustainable. Whether used to complement a broader immune strategy or as a standalone support, beef thymus has clearly left a strong impression on those who needed it most.

Most Reported Benefits from Review Analysis

Beef thymus has earned praise from users seeking to restore energy, improve immune resilience, and support whole-body recovery. With a strong overall customer rating of 4.6 out of 5 stars, it has become a go-to choice for individuals feeling worn down, depleted, or vulnerable to recurring sensitivities. While experiences vary, our analysis of thousands of positive reviews reveals several key patterns that may help you decide whether this supplement aligns with your wellness goals.

The table below highlights the top five benefits most frequently mentioned by users who reported positive outcomes. Each percentage reflects how often a specific benefit was cited among those reviews. A higher percentage suggests that users with similar concerns were more likely to experience support in that area.

For example, if 32% of users who saw improvements mention greater energy, this suggests that energy enhancement is one of the most commonly observed effects. While results may vary, the collective voice of thousands of reviewers offers a meaningful window into what people are actually experiencing.

Below is a summary table of Beef Thymus's top benefits as reported by customers:

Benefit	%	Explanation
Energy Boost	32%	Users frequently describe a surge in stamina, reduced fatigue, and restored vitality, especially during periods of burnout or immune recovery.
Immune Support	27%	Many report fewer seasonal sensitivities, improved immune resilience, and greater overall resistance to environmental triggers.
Healing Support	18%	A wide range of reviews mention improved tissue recovery, faster bounce-back from stress, and support for general system repair.
Infection Defense	13%	Users observed fewer occurrences of common infections and reported feeling more protected during challenging seasons.
Inflammation Relief	10%	Several reviews note a decrease in inflammation-related symptoms such as congestion, skin sensitivity, and joint discomfort.

How to Use This Table

This summary is designed to help you identify whether beef thymus might support your specific needs. The benefits are ranked by how often users experienced them, giving you a realistic picture of what to expect based on the collective experience of others. If you are dealing with low energy, immune imbalance, or lingering recovery issues, this chart may offer insight into how others with similar challenges have responded.

It is important to remember that everyone's body is different. While many users report noticeable improvements, results often depend on factors like dosage consistency, individual sensitivity, and the presence of underlying health issues. Some people notice changes within days, while others observe more gradual shifts over several weeks.

By aligning your expectations with real-world feedback, you can use this guide to better evaluate whether beef thymus may be a supportive addition to your wellness routine.

Beef Brain

Grass-fed beef brain supplements provide a concentrated source of nutrients traditionally associated with cognitive and nervous system support. In ancestral diets, brain tissue was valued for its nutrient density and its potential to nourish the mind and body. Rich in brain-specific peptides, phospholipids, and essential fatty acids, beef brain offers important building blocks that may contribute to neurological health.

Sourced from pasture-raised cattle, beef brain supplements deliver bioavailable compounds such as DHA, phosphatidylserine, and other nutrients linked to memory, nerve support, and mental clarity. For those seeking to support focus, cognitive resilience, or overall brain wellness, beef brain offers a natural, nutrient-dense option worth exploring.

Science-Informed Beef Brain Benefits

Supports Memory and Cognitive Performance

Beef brain contains naturally occurring phosphatidylserine and docosahexaenoic acid (DHA), two important nutrients that play a foundational role in brain cell membrane structure and function. These compounds are involved in maintaining healthy synaptic communication and may contribute to memory formation, attention, and learning capacity. Phosphatidylserine has been studied for its role in supporting executive function, while DHA is known for its role in brain development and cognitive maintenance throughout life. Together, these nutrients help support the overall architecture and signaling mechanisms of the brain.

Many individuals, including students, professionals, and older adults, may consider beef brain as a supplemental option to support clarity of thought, mental stamina, and lifelong cognitive wellness.

Contributes to Nervous System Structure and Repair

Beef brain naturally provides bioactive peptides and molecules such as brain-derived neurotrophic factor (BDNF), which has been studied for its role in supporting neuronal survival, differentiation, and synaptic plasticity. These compounds contribute to the maintenance and adaptability of the nervous system. While the presence of these factors in food-based sources does not guarantee identical physiological effects as those generated internally, they may offer nutritional support for individuals concerned with neurological resilience and nerve health.

This makes beef brain a potentially valuable option for those seeking to support normal nerve function and maintain cognitive integrity under various stressors.

Provides Nutrients Associated with Age-Related Brain Health

As the brain ages, it becomes more vulnerable to oxidative damage and structural decline. Nutrients found in beef brain, including phospholipids, cholesterol, and long-chain omega-3 fatty acids, may help support cellular membrane integrity and reduce oxidative burden. These factors are important for individuals looking to maintain brain vitality during the aging process. While no supplement can prevent or cure neurodegenerative conditions, nutrients that support mitochondrial function and protect cellular membranes may contribute to overall brain resilience.

Beef brain is often considered by individuals who wish to proactively support healthy cognitive aging and protect against age-related decline in mental performance.

Nutritional Support for Mood and Emotional Balance

Beef brain offers essential lipids and amino acids that play roles in the synthesis of neurotransmitters such as serotonin and dopamine. These chemicals help regulate emotional well-being and stress responses. Nutritional cofactors found in brain tissue, including phosphatidylserine and omega-3 fatty acids, may help stabilize mood by supporting the structural components of the brain regions involved in emotional regulation.

Individuals seeking nutritional strategies to support a balanced mood and greater emotional resilience may find beef brain to be a meaningful addition to a comprehensive wellness routine.

May Help Reduce Mental Fatigue and Promote Clarity

DHA is one of the most abundant fatty acids in the brain and plays a key role in maintaining neuronal membrane fluidity, which is important for optimal signal transmission and energy metabolism. Nutritional support from DHA-rich foods, such as beef brain, may contribute to improved mental endurance and focus. Some individuals report greater clarity and reduced fogginess when nutritional gaps are addressed, particularly those involving omega-3 fats and phospholipids.

For those experiencing occasional mental fatigue or seeking to maintain mental alertness throughout the day, beef brain may offer valuable dietary support for sustained brain energy and cognitive clarity.

Customer-Reported Beef Brain Benefits

Beef brain supplements have gained attention among those seeking greater mental clarity, energy, and emotional resilience. With a strong customer satisfaction rating of 4.6 out of 5, many users describe feeling "sharper," "calmer," and more "motivated" after incorporating beef brain into their daily routine. This supplement stands out for its unique nutrient profile, particularly compounds like phosphatidylserine, DHA, and brain-derived peptides, which are believed to support brain cell function and the nervous system.

What sets these reviews apart is not just the positive feedback but the personal transformation many users report. For some, taking beef brain helped lift mental fog that had lingered for years. For others, it restored a sense of purpose, allowing them to tackle projects, connect more deeply with loved ones, or return to activities they once enjoyed. The emotional tone ranges from quiet gratitude to outright amazement, often expressing disbelief at how such a simple addition made a meaningful difference.

Let's explore how users most commonly describe the benefits they experienced.

Use Case Patterns Observed

Many people turn to beef brain to support memory, focus, and emotional balance. A common pattern includes individuals seeking support for age-related memory lapses, stress-related brain fog, or general mental sluggishness. Some report using it to help recover from emotional or neurological stress, while others incorporate it into protocols for mood or nervous system support. A notable number of users mention benefits related to motivation, productivity, and the ability to complete everyday tasks, whether planning finances, returning to hobbies, or organizing personal projects.

Parents have also shared stories of using beef brain to support their children's focus and development, often mixing capsules into food. Others use it during times of high cognitive demand, such as during fasting, exams, or emotionally intense periods. Users with demanding mental workloads, teachers, healthcare professionals, IT workers, and veterans, are particularly likely to report noticeable improvements in clarity and task management. Some also mention taking beef brain alongside other organ-based supplements like liver, heart, or bone marrow to create a more holistic nutritional foundation.

Feedback Insights

The emotional tone in customer feedback is both sincere and striking. Many express deep relief at finally feeling "awake" again after years of mental fog. One reviewer described the change as a "light switch flipping on" in their brain, while another shared that they could finally read decades-old family letters, something they had put off for years due to mental fatigue. Users describe their thoughts as clearer, more organized, and easier to follow. Several note a renewed ability to recall details, complete tasks without procrastination, or handle emotionally complex situations with greater calm.

For some, the improvements extend beyond cognitive performance into emotional resilience. Users frequently mention feeling more centered, emotionally steady, or peaceful. A few even describe the experience as life-changing, particularly those who had previously felt overwhelmed, detached, or discouraged by ongoing brain fog, mood swings, or nervous tension. One reviewer noted, "I can joke more, goof off more, and be more playful with my kids," while another said, "I remembered my dreams for the first time in years."

There are also heartfelt expressions of hope and renewed identity. Individuals who had struggled with cognitive decline or emotional fatigue feeling that they had regained a part of themselves. Whether helping people prepare for meetings, face difficult seasons, or simply feel more "present" in their day, beef brain has earned praise as a supplement that quietly but powerfully supports mental and emotional well-being.

Most Reported Benefits from Review Analysis

Beef brain supplements have drawn widespread attention from users seeking better focus, sharper thinking, and renewed energy. With an impressive customer satisfaction rating of 4.6 out of 5 stars, many people describe a noticeable shift in how they feel mentally and emotionally, reporting everything from enhanced concentration and improved memory to a sense of feeling "clear" and "alive" again.

To better understand these outcomes, we analyzed thousands of verified customer reviews and identified the most commonly reported benefits. These figures reflect how often each benefit was mentioned by users who had a positive experience. A higher percentage suggests that more users noticed that specific outcome.

For example, if 35 percent of reviewers mentioned improved energy, that indicates a high likelihood that others with similar concerns may also feel more energized or mentally alert. While individual results will always vary, this feedback offers meaningful guidance when considering how beef brain might fit into your own routine.

Below is a summary table of Beef Brain's top benefits as reported by customers:

Benefit	%	Explanation
Energy boost	35%	Many users report a significant increase in both mental and physical energy, helping them stay sharp and engaged throughout the day.
Focus improvement	21%	Users often describe enhanced concentration and improved attention span, which supports better performance in both work and daily tasks.
Mental clarity	17%	A noticeable return of mental sharpness, with users saying they can think more clearly and feel less scattered.
Brain fog relief	15%	Many reviewers experience a reduction in cognitive haze, reporting it's easier to think quickly and stay mentally present.
Memory support	13%	Users note improvements in short-term and long-term memory, including better recall of names, tasks, and past events.

How to Use This Table

This table provides a snapshot of the most frequently reported outcomes among satisfied users. If you see a benefit that aligns with what you are currently experiencing, such as low energy, difficulty focusing, or mental fog, those higher percentages may signal a stronger potential match for your needs. While not every person experiences every benefit, this kind of real-world data can help guide expectations and highlight how others have found value in incorporating beef brain into their health routine.

Beef Collagen

Beef collagen, derived from grass-fed bovine sources, is one of the most trusted and effective supplements for supporting structural health from the inside out. As the most abundant protein in the body, collagen is essential for maintaining the integrity of skin, joints, bones, tendons, and connective tissues. With age, natural collagen production declines, leading to visible signs of aging, joint stiffness, brittle nails, and thinning hair. Beef collagen replenishes the body's supply with highly bioavailable peptides that restore, protect, and strengthen tissues throughout the body.

Unlike topical creams or short-term solutions, collagen supplementation works at the foundational level to rebuild the body's natural scaffolding. Rich in amino acids like glycine, proline, and hydroxyproline, beef collagen helps promote skin elasticity, joint mobility, and overall vitality. Whether your goal is to reduce joint pain, improve skin appearance, strengthen hair and nails, or simply age more gracefully, beef collagen offers a powerful way to renew and fortify your body from within.

Science-Informed Beef Collagen Benefits

Beef collagen, sourced from grass-fed bovine, provides a concentrated supply of type I and type III collagen, the two most prevalent forms found in the human body. These structural proteins are essential for the integrity of skin, joints, bones, muscles, and connective tissues. Over time, natural collagen production declines, which can affect the body's resilience and flexibility. Supplementing with high-quality beef collagen offers a way to support the body's ongoing need for these foundational proteins.

Supports Joint Structure and Mobility

Collagen is a central component of joint cartilage, contributing to its strength, elasticity, and ability to cushion movement. As cartilage wears down over time or due to mechanical stress, mobility may be affected. Beef collagen provides amino acids that are necessary for maintaining cartilage health and joint function. Emerging studies suggest that collagen peptides may play a supportive role in physical performance and comfort during movement, especially in aging populations or those with physically demanding lifestyles.

Promotes Skin Structure and Moisture Retention

The dermis layer of the skin is composed primarily of collagen, which helps maintain firmness and elasticity. As collagen levels decline, the skin may gradually lose moisture and resilience. Supplementing with bovine collagen has been studied for its ability to support skin hydration, smoothness, and elasticity. These benefits appear to be linked to collagen's role in encouraging the body's own production of new collagen and its interaction with other skin-supportive compounds like hyaluronic acid.

Contributes to Hair and Nail Strength

Beef collagen is rich in proline and glycine, amino acids involved in the synthesis of keratin, the key structural protein in both hair and nails. By supporting the nutritional environment for keratin formation, collagen may contribute to stronger, more resilient hair strands and reduced brittleness in nails. Users seeking to maintain the appearance and strength of these features often include collagen as part of a broader nutritional approach to personal care.

Supports Bone Matrix and Mineralization

Collagen acts as the internal framework of bone tissue, giving bones their flexibility and shape before mineral components are laid down. As collagen declines with age, bones can become more fragile. Research has shown that collagen supplementation may help support the activity of bone-forming cells and maintain structural density when paired with essential nutrients like calcium and vitamin D. This makes collagen a valuable addition to a comprehensive approach to skeletal health.

Aids Muscle Recovery and Tissue Repair

Collagen contains amino acids such as glycine and arginine that are important for muscle protein synthesis and connective tissue strength. These compounds also contribute to creatine production, which supports energy availability in muscle cells. When combined with strength training, collagen supplementation has been associated with positive changes in body composition, including increased lean mass and enhanced post-exercise recovery. These benefits are thought to stem from collagen's role in maintaining tendon and ligament health alongside muscle tissue.

Customer-Reported Beef Collagen Benefits

Collagen is one of the most abundant proteins in the human body, yet many people do not realize how deeply it influences the health and function of skin, joints, hair, nails, and even digestion. As natural collagen production declines with age, many turn to beef collagen supplements in search of support for aging skin, creaky joints, and brittle nails. Among those who regularly take beef collagen, the sense of renewal is often described as both visible and deeply felt. From smoother skin to more flexible joints, the reported benefits extend across many areas of physical wellness. With an impressive average rating of 4.7 out of 5 stars across thousands of reviews, this supplement has made a noticeable impact for many individuals seeking natural, structural support.

Use Case Patterns Observed

People reach for beef collagen supplements for a wide variety of reasons, often related to the visible or physical signs of aging. A large portion of users begin taking it for support with joint stiffness, mobility concerns, or discomfort in the knees, back, or hands. Others are motivated by a desire to improve skin quality, reduce the appearance of wrinkles, or boost elasticity. Many individuals also report trying collagen to strengthen weak nails, thicken thinning hair, or reduce excessive shedding. Some have switched from powdered products to capsules for convenience, especially those with digestive sensitivities or busy schedules. Athletes, active professionals, and older adults frequently take beef collagen as part of a broader effort to support recovery, maintain mobility, and preserve their quality of life as they age.

Feedback Insights

The emotional language used in reviews often reflects a deep sense of gratitude and personal transformation. Many people describe being "amazed" by the difference they noticed in their hair, nails, or skin within just a few weeks. One user wrote that her skin became "soft, hydrated, and supple" after consistent use, while another commented, "It's like I'm wearing foundation, but I'm not." Joints were also a common theme. Numerous reviewers reported feeling more limber, with several noting that joint discomfort they had lived with for years had eased significantly. Phrases like "I can finally move without pain," or "My knees feel better than they have in years," were frequent. Some even mentioned feeling more confident and youthful, with comments such as "People say I look younger," and "I feel stronger and more energized every day."

The changes were not only visible but often deeply encouraging. For many, stronger nails and shinier hair became symbolic of inner renewal. One reviewer shared that she saw baby hairs growing in spots where she previously had thinning, calling it "nothing short of incredible." Even those who were initially skeptical or had tried other products in the past described this collagen as "the only one that actually worked." Others mentioned that the improvement in skin tone or joint comfort helped them return to exercise or enjoy everyday activities more fully.

Most Reported Benefits from Review Analysis

Beef collagen has become one of the most widely praised supplements for those seeking support with beauty, mobility, and everyday vitality. With an impressive average rating of 4.7 out of 5 from tens of thousands of users, many report noticeable improvements in skin, joints, hair, and nails. These real-world results have made beef collagen a go-to choice for individuals looking for both visible and internal support as they age or maintain an active lifestyle.

Our analysis of thousands of positive reviews reveals which benefits are mentioned most frequently by users who experienced meaningful results. Each review was evaluated for specific outcomes, and every mentioned benefit was counted individually, even when a review listed more than one. This method provides a clear picture of the benefits people most often associate with beef collagen supplementation.

For instance, if 28 percent of positive reviews mention improvements in skin health, that means more than one in four satisfied users specifically noticed changes in skin hydration, firmness, or appearance.

Below is a summary table of beef collagen's top benefits as reported by customers:

Benefit	%	Explanation
Skin health	28%	A noticeable improvement in skin hydration, elasticity, and radiance. Users frequently report firmer, smoother, and more youthful-looking skin with fewer fine lines or dry patches.
Joint comfort	25%	Relief from joint discomfort and stiffness. Many users feel more mobile and physically at ease during exercise, work, or daily movement after taking collagen consistently.
Hair health	24%	Reports of thicker, shinier, and faster-growing hair. Reviewers frequently mention reduced shedding and improved strength, especially after hair loss or thinning.
Nail strength	17%	Nails become stronger and more resistant to breaking or peeling. Many users see faster growth and healthier nail appearance within a few weeks.
Gut health	5%	A smaller group of users mention better digestion, less bloating, or a more comfortable gut experience, potentially due to collagen's naturally occurring amino acids.

How to Use This Table

These percentages reflect how often each benefit was mentioned by users who shared positive results. They are not clinical findings, but they do provide insight into what people commonly notice when taking beef collagen. If your goals align with one or more of the benefits listed above, you may find this supplement especially relevant. As with any health product, individual experiences vary, and results often depend on consistent use and lifestyle factors.

Taken together, these real-world responses show that beef collagen is valued for its ability to support the way people look, move, and feel. Whether you are seeking smoother skin, stronger joints, better hair and nails, or gentle digestive support, many users have found beef collagen to be a helpful addition to their wellness routine.

Beef Cartilage

Beef cartilage, such as that found in beef trachea, is a traditional whole-food source of nutrients long valued for supporting joint and connective tissue health. Derived from grass-fed cattle, beef cartilage provides naturally occurring compounds like collagen type II, chondroitin sulfate, glucosamine, and hyaluronic acid, nutrients that contribute to joint lubrication, cartilage integrity, and structural resilience.

In traditional cultures, cartilage-rich foods like bone marrow, joints, and trachea were regularly consumed as part of a diet intended to support physical strength and mobility over time. Today, modern interest has returned to these ancestral practices, recognizing that whole-food cartilage may provide a concentrated and bioavailable source of key building blocks for the musculoskeletal system.

For individuals seeking nutritional support for joint comfort, structural balance, and connective tissue nourishment, beef cartilage offers a natural way to reinforce the body's foundation and support healthy movement.

Science-Informed Beef Cartilage Benefits

Supports Cartilage Structure and Joint Integrity

Beef cartilage is particularly rich in type II collagen, the form of collagen most prevalent in joint cartilage. This protein forms the structural framework of cartilage and plays a central role in maintaining its tensile strength and resilience. Nutritionally supporting the body's supply of type II collagen may help reinforce cartilage over time, especially in areas subject to repetitive movement or load-bearing activity. By delivering a direct source of structural components, beef cartilage may contribute to the natural maintenance of healthy joint tissue.

Provides Nutrients Associated with Joint Comfort and Mobility

Beef cartilage is a natural source of chondroitin sulfate and glucosamine, two well-studied compounds commonly found in connective tissues. These nutrients are known for their roles in supporting joint cushioning and promoting normal inflammatory responses. While individual experiences vary, some studies suggest that regular intake of chondroitin and glucosamine may help maintain comfort during movement, particularly in physically active individuals or those experiencing age-related stiffness. Consuming cartilage as a whole-food supplement provides these compounds in a naturally occurring matrix that may enhance their bioavailability.

Contributes to Joint Lubrication and Smooth Movement

One of the most important compounds found in beef cartilage is hyaluronic acid, a naturally occurring substance that helps retain moisture within joint spaces. By attracting and holding water inside the joint capsule, hyaluronic acid supports the lubrication that allows for smooth and flexible motion. Nutritional support for hyaluronic acid levels may be especially beneficial for knees, hips, shoulders, and other joints where daily activity or aging can reduce fluid volume and affect comfort.

Nourishes the Connective Tissue Network

Beyond joint cartilage, beef cartilage provides structural nutrients that benefit a wide range of connective tissues, including tendons, ligaments, fascia, and even intervertebral discs. The unique combination of amino acids, collagen peptides, and glycosaminoglycans found in cartilage contributes to the body's ability to maintain tissue integrity and elasticity. This type of nutritional support is often sought out by individuals who are physically active, recovering from strain, or aiming to support long-term flexibility and tissue resilience.

Explored for Immune and Gut-Related Benefits

Early research into undenatured type II collagen, a form preserved in some cartilage preparations, suggests it may influence immune signaling pathways when taken orally. Some scientists are exploring its potential role in promoting immune system balance by reducing over-reactivity to self-tissues. This has led to growing interest in its possible applications for gut-joint interactions and broader systemic wellness. While more studies are needed, these early findings highlight a promising area of research into the immune-modulating potential of beef cartilage.

Customer-Reported Beef Cartilage Benefits

Beef cartilage has earned strong praise from individuals seeking natural support for joint health, tissue recovery, and structural resilience. With an average rating of 4.6 out of 5, reviewers consistently report meaningful improvements in flexibility, reduced discomfort, and increased energy and mobility. Many describe a noticeable change in how their bodies feel, especially in areas affected by long-term wear, aging, or past injuries.

Our review analysis identified patterns in how users describe their experiences and what benefits they report most often. Each mention of a benefit, such as joint comfort or skin improvement, was counted separately, even if a reviewer noted several outcomes. This approach reveals which benefits are most frequently experienced among those who reported positive results.

Use Case Patterns Observed

Beef cartilage supplements are most commonly used by individuals experiencing joint stiffness, past injuries, or chronic musculoskeletal discomfort. Many reviewers specifically mention using it after trying other solutions, including over-the-counter pain relievers or prescription medications. Others report using it alongside complementary supplements such as collagen, bone marrow, or organ blends to create a more comprehensive approach to physical recovery and performance.

Among the most prominent user groups are adults with age-related joint wear, athletes and active individuals recovering from strain or injury, and those with connective tissue or autoimmune conditions affecting soft tissue health. A smaller number also mention using it for skin vitality, energy, and structural support during intensive physical demands or health recovery processes.

Several reviews highlight use by both humans and pets, especially older dogs with mobility challenges, suggesting a wide trust in its bioavailable support across different health needs.

Feedback Insights

Reviewers frequently describe a deep sense of gratitude and even surprise at how much better they feel after incorporating beef cartilage into their routine. Many express relief at being able to move more freely, noting that persistent stiffness, swelling, or cracking in their knees, hips, or back noticeably decreased. Phrases such as "pain-free again," "mobility is back," and "I can move without aching" appear repeatedly, showing how significant even small improvements can feel to those dealing with chronic discomfort.

Others report being "astounded" or "impressed" by the level of difference the supplement made, especially when used alongside collagen or bone and marrow. Emotional language like "life-changing," "finally found something that works," and "so thankful I discovered this" reflects how personally meaningful these improvements are to users who had tried other approaches with limited results.

In addition to physical benefits, some describe an unexpected boost in energy, mood, or sense of well-being. A few even note clearer skin or improved recovery after illness or surgery, pointing to its wider impact on tissue integrity and immune resilience.

Many reviewers also express a strong connection to the product's ancestral, whole-food sourcing. Several mention they feel more confident and grounded using natural supplements that align with how the body evolved to heal and rebuild.

Most Reported Benefits from Review Analysis

Beef cartilage, often sourced from beef trachea, has become a well-recognized choice for those seeking natural support for joint comfort, cartilage regeneration, and long-term mobility. With an impressive average rating of 4.6 out of 5, this supplement has gained widespread praise from users who describe meaningful improvements in how their joints feel and function. Whether dealing with age-related stiffness, injury recovery, or persistent joint discomfort, many individuals turn to beef cartilage for targeted, whole-food support.

Our analysis of thousands of positive customer reviews reveals which benefits are mentioned most frequently among those who experienced results. Each mention was counted independently, even when reviewers listed multiple benefits in the same comment. This method helps highlight which outcomes stand out most across a wide range of users.

For example, if 53% of positive reviews reference joint pain relief, that means more than half of satisfied users specifically noticed improvements in that area.

Below is a summary of the top customer-validated benefits of beef cartilage:

Benefit	%	Explanation
Joint Pain / Joint Support	53%	Many users report less joint pain, better comfort, and increased joint stability during daily movement.
Cartilage Repair / Regeneration	16%	Users describe greater resilience in worn-down joints, with some noticing visible recovery over time.
Knee Pain	16%	Common reports of reduced knee discomfort and better function when walking, climbing stairs, or exercising.
Flexibility / Mobility	8%	Reviewers often mention smoother movement, less stiffness, and greater ease during physical activity.
Back Pain / Spine Support	6%	A smaller but notable group describe reduced discomfort in the lower back and better spinal alignment.

How to Use This Table

This table summarizes the most frequently reported benefits among users who had a positive experience with beef cartilage. The percentages reflect how often each benefit was mentioned in successful outcomes. A higher percentage suggests that users with similar concerns may be more likely to notice results in that area. While individual responses vary, this real-world insight can help guide your expectations and support your decision-making process as you explore natural options for joint and tissue support.

With consistently strong reviews and a clear trend in user-reported outcomes, beef cartilage continues to stand out as a trusted supplement for those seeking comfort, strength, and flexibility through whole-food nourishment.

Beef Organs for
Everyday Health Goals

Earlier chapters introduced each beef organ supplement individually, exploring their science-informed properties and the most commonly reported user experiences. This chapter shifts the lens: it organizes those insights by health goals, making it easier for you to explore which organ supplements are most frequently associated with specific areas of wellness such as energy, hormone balance, skin health, or joint comfort.

The percentages listed next to each organ reflect data from our *Most Reported Benefits from Review Analysis*, a method that examines thousands of real-world user reviews to identify the most frequently mentioned benefits. These numbers show how often a specific outcome was mentioned relative to other effects, offering a practical snapshot of how people are using these supplements in everyday life.

This chapter is not meant to replace the detailed organ profiles shared earlier, but rather to provide a user-friendly reference guide. It offers a clear, high-level overview to help you match your health goals with the organs that may be worth considering, based on a blend of science-informed knowledge and real-world patterns.

Please remember that the insights shared here are not medical advice and are not intended to diagnose, treat, or cure any condition. While many people report positive experiences, results can vary based on individual health, habits, and consistency of use. Natural supplements do not guarantee specific outcomes.

This chapter is here to help you make thoughtful, informed choices on your wellness journey. If you are considering organ-based supplements as part of your health plan, these insights may offer a useful starting point to explore in partnership with a qualified healthcare professional.

Blood and Circulatory Wellness

Spleen (40%) – Iron and Hemoglobin Support. Users frequently report improved iron status and fewer symptoms associated with iron deficiency, such as dizziness and fatigue. Scientific studies suggest that spleen tissue may support red blood cell maintenance and the body's natural iron recycling process. Nutrients in spleen are also involved in regulating iron stores and hemoglobin synthesis.

Spleen (23%) – Red Blood Cell and Circulatory Function. Often chosen for its potential to support healthy red blood cell turnover and circulation, contributing to overall stamina and vitality. Scientific literature indicates that spleen extracts may help reinforce blood filtration and red blood cell integrity.

Respiratory and Seasonal Comfort

Lung (50%) – Breathing and Lung Function. Many users describe easier breathing, improved respiratory comfort, and enhanced endurance during daily activities. Scientific studies suggest that nutrients in lung tissue may help nourish respiratory structures and promote efficient oxygen exchange.

Lung (14%) – Respiratory Resilience. Individuals managing chronic respiratory challenges often report noticeable improvement.

Preliminary research has explored the potential of lung-specific peptides to support airway comfort and reduce respiratory stress.

Bone, Joint and Muscle Support

Bone and Skeletal Strength

Bone and Marrow (12%) – Skeletal Support. Many users report improved bone strength and greater resilience. Research indicates that bone marrow is a natural source of minerals and collagen that help maintain bone density and structural integrity.

Joint Comfort and Mobility Support

Cartilage (61%) – Joint Comfort and Mobility. Users frequently mention noticeable relief from joint discomfort and enhanced flexibility. These reports are especially common among older adults and those with joint sensitivity. Scientific findings support the role of type II collagen and glycosaminoglycans (GAGs) from beef cartilage in supporting joint structure, lubrication, and healthy inflammation response.

Collagen (25%) – Joint Comfort. Often chosen for its ability to ease stiffness and discomfort during movement. Research shows that naturally occurring collagen may help maintain elasticity and cushioning in joint tissues.

Cartilage (16%) – Knee Support. Many individuals with knee sensitivity report easier movement and reduced pain in daily tasks. Research suggests that compounds in cartilage, including chondroitin sulfate, may support comfort and mobility in weight-bearing joints.

Bone and Marrow (17%) – Joint Function. Users often note smoother motion and less stiffness, particularly in aging joints. Studies have linked bone marrow-derived compounds to natural support for cartilage and joint lubrication.

Cartilage (16%) – Cartilage Structure. Some users report gradual improvements in areas of long-standing cartilage strain. Scientific research supports the potential role of undenatured type II collagen in promoting cartilage integrity and supporting the body's natural repair pathways.

Bone and Marrow (10%) – Cartilage Support. Selected for its potential to aid flexibility and joint resilience. Bioactive compounds in bone marrow are associated with connective tissue repair and joint maintenance.

Muscle Function

Testicles (19%) – Muscle and Recovery Support. Commonly used by physically active individuals seeking better muscle tone and endurance. Scientific sources indicate that testicular extracts may contain natural precursors that help support muscle maintenance and energy production.

Immune System Support

Thymus (40%) – Immune Function and Seasonal Defense. Many users report feeling more resilient during seasonal changes and note fewer sick days. Scientific studies suggest that thymic peptides help regulate T-cell activity and support a balanced immune response.

Thymus (28%) – Recovery and Inflammatory Balance. Often used by individuals recovering from physical stress, procedures, or inflammation-related concerns. Research indicates that thymic compounds may support tissue repair and help modulate inflammatory markers in the body.

Colostrum (16%) – Natural Immune Support. Commonly chosen for its contribution to immune preparedness, especially in high-exposure environments. Scientific evidence shows that colostrum contains immunoglobulins and growth factors that play a role in strengthening natural defenses.

Kidney (26%) – Histamine and Sensitivity Balance. Users with occasional sensitivity to foods or environmental factors often report fewer discomforts. Scientific studies suggest that kidney tissue may contain diamine oxidase (DAO), an enzyme involved in histamine breakdown and balance.

Hormonal and Reproductive Wellness

Female Organs (17%) – Cycle and Hormonal Rhythm Support. Individuals report more consistent menstrual cycles and improved comfort. Scientific literature indicates that nutrients in female reproductive tissue may contain hormone precursors that contribute to hormonal regulation.

Female Organs (15%) – Emotional and Mood Stability. Many users describe a sense of emotional balance and steadier mood throughout the month. Scientific studies support that compounds found in these tissues may influence hormonal equilibrium.

Testicles (9%) – Androgen Support and Vitality. Users commonly report better overall energy and motivation. Research suggests that testicular extracts contain androgens and related nutrients that may help support testosterone balance.

Testicles (9%) – Physical Strength and Endurance. Particularly among active individuals, many report enhanced stamina and post-exercise recovery. Studies show that testosterone is involved in muscle repair and physical performance.

Cognitive Clarity and Mental Performance

Brain (32%) – Mental Sharpness and Clarity. Many individuals note a clearer mind and reduced cognitive fatigue. Research suggests that neurotrophic compounds in brain tissue may help support neuron signaling and mental clarity.

Brain (30%) – Concentration and Focus. Users often report increased focus and productivity. Scientific sources indicate that brain-derived phospholipids and peptides may play a role in sustaining attention and mental stamina.

Brain (23%) – Memory and Cognitive Support. Many report better recall, faster thinking, and enhanced mental agility. Studies highlight that neuropeptides found in brain extracts support memory-related brain function.

Thyroid (10%) – Mental Energy and Cognitive Support. Especially noted by those with thyroid-related sluggishness, users describe better clarity and mental function. Scientific research confirms that healthy thyroid function is crucial for supporting brain activity and mental alertness.

Digestive & Gastrointestinal Health

Pancreas (78%) – Digestive Function and Gut Comfort. Users often report reduced bloating, improved digestion, and better tolerance of meals. Scientific research shows that pancreatic enzymes play a vital role in breaking down fats, proteins, and carbohydrates, which supports digestive efficiency and relief from upper GI discomfort.

Pancreas (21%) – Pancreatic Health. Many individuals choose this supplement to help maintain normal pancreatic function and digestive enzyme balance. Scientific studies suggest that extracts from pancreatic tissue may support the body's enzyme activity and metabolic regulation.

Colostrum (25%) – Gut Barrier and Microbiome Support. Users describe improved digestive comfort, fewer issues with bloating, and better overall gut function. Scientific evidence shows that immunoglobulins in colostrum help maintain gut lining integrity and support microbiome balance.

Colostrum (12%) – Digestive Efficiency. Some users report easier digestion and less stomach sensitivity. Research suggests that the growth factors in colostrum may help support gut lining health and nutrient absorption.

Energy & Vitality

Female Organs (60%) – Daily Energy and Mood Resilience. Many users note a noticeable increase in daily vitality, clarity, and emotional balance. Scientific literature indicates that female organ tissues may contain hormone precursors that help support energy regulation and overall well-being.

Testicles (56%) – Physical Stamina and Performance. Users often report better endurance, workout recovery, and sustained physical output. Scientific studies suggest that testicular extracts provide nutrients and androgens that may play a role in supporting energy metabolism.

Organs Blend (62%) – Overall Vitality. This multi-organ blend is commonly praised for improving general energy and motivation. Scientific research indicates that the wide nutrient profile in these blends may support cellular energy production and systemic function.

Bone and Marrow (37%) – Physical Strength and Endurance. Users frequently describe enhanced strength during daily tasks and improved stamina. Studies highlight that bone marrow provides essential nutrients like iron and collagen that support oxygen transport and musculoskeletal energy.

Liver (46%) – Alertness and Reduced Fatigue. Individuals report increased clarity and reduced sluggishness. Scientific research shows that liver is a rich source of B vitamins, iron, and CoQ10, all of which are central to mitochondrial energy production.

Brain (35%) – Mental Energy and Drive. Many users experience a boost in both cognitive sharpness and motivation. Studies suggest that phospholipids and neurotrophic compounds found in brain tissue may help support neurological energy balance.

Thymus (32%) – Steady Daily Energy. Users describe a more even energy flow throughout the day with fewer crashes. Research suggests thymic peptides may help support immune and metabolic balance, contributing to overall energy stability.

Thyroid (28%) – Metabolic Energy Support. Users with low thyroid function often report increased energy and mental clarity. Scientific evidence confirms that thyroid hormones play a crucial role in mitochondrial function and metabolism.

Spleen (27%) – Oxygenation and Stamina. Individuals managing low iron or fatigue note improved energy over time. Scientific studies support the spleen's role in red blood cell turnover and healthy circulation, which supports oxygen delivery.

Adrenal (35%) – Adrenal Energy and Stress Resilience. Commonly used by individuals with chronic fatigue, this supplement is praised for helping to stabilize energy. Research suggests adrenal tissue extracts may influence cortisol balance and energy regulation.

Stress and Emotional Balance

Adrenal (55%) – Stress Resilience and Emotional Stability. Many users report feeling calmer, more balanced, and less overwhelmed during times of pressure or fatigue. Scientific studies show that adrenal extracts contain compounds involved in the body's natural stress response, including hormone precursors that influence mood, resilience, and energy regulation.

Sleep Quality

Adrenal (10%) – Sleep Rhythm and Restfulness. Some users note more restful and uninterrupted sleep patterns. Research indicates that adrenal-related hormone balance may play a role in supporting circadian stability and nighttime relaxation.

Thyroid (10%) – Sleep Quality in Low Thyroid Function. Individuals managing thyroid imbalances report more ease falling and staying asleep. Scientific studies suggest that optimal thyroid hormone levels are associated with improved sleep quality and duration.

Urinary and Kidney Wellness

Kidney (44%) – Renal Function and Urinary Comfort. Users frequently report reduced bloating and more regular urination. Scientific research highlights that kidney extracts may contain peptides and nutrients that contribute to renal tissue nourishment and fluid balance.

Metabolic Support

Thyroid (15%) – Metabolic Activity and Weight Regulation. Users often describe improvements in metabolic energy and steady weight support. Scientific literature confirms that thyroid hormones are essential for regulating metabolic rate and energy expenditure.

Pancreas (12%) – Glucose and Energy Stability. Many users report steadier energy levels and improved carbohydrate tolerance. Studies suggest that pancreatic extracts may help support enzymatic function and blood sugar regulation.

Cardiovascular and Circulatory Wellness

Heart (57%) – Cardiovascular Strength and Endurance. Users report enhanced stamina, circulation, and physical output. Research shows that heart tissue provides nutrients like CoQ10 and essential amino acids that support cardiac muscle and overall heart function.

Heart (12%) – Circulatory Balance. Some users describe more consistent blood pressure readings. Scientific findings indicate that heart extracts may help support vascular tone and circulatory health.

Skin, Hair and Nail Health

Skin Wellness

Collagen (28%) – Hydration, Firmness, and Appearance. Users frequently report smoother, firmer, and more radiant skin. Scientific studies suggest that collagen peptides support dermal density and promote fibroblast activity for visible skin health.

Bone and Marrow (24%) – Elasticity and Moisture Balance. Many individuals notice improved skin tone and hydration. Research shows that bone marrow is rich in collagen-boosting nutrients that support the skin's structural foundation.

Organs Blend (22%) – Texture and Irritation Relief. Users commonly report a decrease in dryness and blemishes. Scientific evidence supports that blended organ nutrients contribute to skin balance through a wide range of vitamins and minerals.

Colostrum (22%) – Skin Calm and Clarity. Users describe smoother, clearer skin and reduced irritation. Research shows that colostrum contains compounds that may help calm skin inflammation and support tissue recovery.

Liver (18%) – Complexion and Detox Support. Individuals often experience a clearer, more even complexion. Studies confirm that liver is a potent source of vitamin A and detoxification cofactors that contribute to skin renewal.

Thymus (18%) – Skin Flare-Ups and Immune Balance. Some users managing skin sensitivity or reactivity report visible improvements. Scientific findings suggest thymic peptides may influence immune pathways connected to skin inflammation.

Hair Health Support

Collagen (24%) – Hair Strength and Growth. Users commonly report shinier, thicker hair with less breakage. Studies support that collagen provides key amino acids that nourish hair follicles and aid keratin production.

Liver (21%) – Shine and Fullness. Many users notice fuller, more vibrant hair. Scientific studies show liver is rich in iron, biotin, and vitamin A, nutrients linked to healthy scalp and hair growth.

Organs Blend (12%) – Overall Hair Nourishment. Users report reduced shedding and improved texture. Research indicates that nutrient-diverse organ blends may support hair vitality by supplying critical building blocks.

Nail Strength and Growth

Collagen (17%) – Nail Growth and Thickness. Users frequently report longer, stronger nails with fewer chips or breaks. Scientific findings suggest that collagen supports nail density and keratin structure.

Liver (15%) – Nail Durability and Smoothness. Individuals with brittle or fragile nails note clear improvement. Research shows that liver supplies micronutrients like zinc, iron, and B vitamins critical for nail strength and resilience.

Practical Applications
of Animal Organ Therapy

Grass-fed beef (and other animal-derived) organ supplements offer a natural, whole-food source of essential nutrients that help maintain the healthy function of vital systems in the body. Rich in vitamins, minerals, and bioactive compounds, these supplements provide a convenient way to consume the nutritional benefits of organ meats without the need for cooking or preparation. Available in capsule or powder form, they can easily fit into busy modern routines.

Convenient Capsule Use

Capsules are one of the most accessible ways to take beef organ supplements. They are portable, pre-measured, and eliminate the need to prepare or cook organ meats. For those who prefer not to swallow capsules, the contents can be opened and mixed into soft foods or drinks. This flexible use still delivers the same concentrated nutritional profile in a form that works for different preferences and needs.

Dosage Recommendations and Gradual Introduction

Most organ supplements include suggested usage instructions on the label, which are generally intended for maintenance and wellness. For personalized use or specific health goals, consulting with a knowledgeable healthcare provider is always advisable.

A gradual approach is often recommended: start with 1 capsule daily and increase by 1 capsule every 2 to 3 days until reaching the full recommended serving. This slow introduction allows the body to adjust and helps identify the optimal dose for individual comfort.

Pay attention to how you feel as you increase your dose. While some individuals thrive on smaller amounts, others may benefit from a full daily serving. Adjust your intake based on energy, digestion, and overall well-being.

Best Timing for Use

Beef organ supplements are derived from whole-food sources and can be taken with or without food at any time of day. However, some people may find they feel more energized after taking them. To avoid any potential disruption to sleep, many prefer to take them in the morning or early afternoon for steady energy throughout the day.

Safety and Precautions

Organ supplements are considered safe for most individuals when used as directed. However, it's important to keep the following in mind:

Health Conditions: Individuals with pre-existing health conditions should consult a qualified healthcare professional before adding new supplements to their routine.

Pregnancy and Breastfeeding: It is advisable to consult with a practitioner before using any organ supplements during pregnancy or while nursing.

Dosage Awareness: Avoid exceeding the recommended amount. Even natural, whole-food supplements may lead to discomfort or unwanted effects when taken in excess.

A Final Word:
The Journey to Vibrant Health

As we come to the end of this journey through Animal Organ Therapy, it's worth reflecting on the power and simplicity of what you've explored. The supplements and principles introduced in this book are not quick fixes, but time-tested, nature-based tools that many have found helpful in supporting their health and vitality.

Throughout these pages, you've discovered how organ-based nutrition may complement your wellness goals, whether you're seeking to feel more energized, support a specific body system, or maintain long-term vitality. Grounded in both scientific insight and real-world experience, Animal Organ Therapy offers a practical and thoughtful path forward.

What makes this approach especially powerful is how accessible it is. You don't need to dramatically change your lifestyle to begin. For many, simply incorporating one or two high-quality organ supplements into a daily routine becomes an easy, effective way to nourish the body from within. Taken in capsule or powder form, these nutrients can be seamlessly integrated into even the busiest lives.

This book is not the end of your journey; it's a starting point. Natural wellness is not about chasing perfection, but about building consistency, honoring your body's needs, and staying open to simple practices that work in harmony with your system. Every small step, whether it's taking a supplement, listening to your body, or making mindful choices, adds up over time.

The Medicine-Free, Illness-Free Series is here to walk with you on that path. Other volumes explore Herbal Therapy, Mushroom Therapy, Amino Acid Therapy, the HOPED Protocol, Detoxification Therapy, Grounding Therapy, and Diet, Lifestyle, and Emotional Well-being, each offering science-informed, user-friendly guidance to help you make empowered health decisions.

May this book inspire you to continue your journey with confidence and curiosity. Your body holds remarkable wisdom. With the right support, vibrant health is not only possible, it's within reach.

To explore more natural solutions or receive personalized guidance, visit AshiHealing.com.

About the Author

Dr. Forest Yin (Jie Yin) is a licensed acupuncturist, herbalist, and Doctor of Acupuncture and Oriental Medicine (DAOM). He serves as a professor and doctoral advisor at the University of East West Medicine (UEWM) and is the founder of Ashi Healing and Acupuncture Inc. With extensive experience in Traditional Chinese Medicine (TCM) and natural health, Dr. Yin integrates a wide range of holistic therapies, forming the foundation of *The Medicine-Free, Illness-Free Series*.

Before devoting his career fully to natural healing, Dr. Yin worked in the high-tech and financial sectors with both large corporations and fast-paced startups. These experiences gave him firsthand insight into the chronic stress and burnout common in modern life. Inspired to seek sustainable strategies for long-term wellness, he turned to the wisdom of nature and the depth of Chinese medicine.

Dr. Yin's clinical experience and ongoing research have helped shape practical wellness protocols that focus on balance, energy, and lifestyle-based health support. His work emphasizes simple, science-informed approaches that align with the body's natural rhythms and support overall resilience.

Driven by a mission to empower others, he created *The Medicine-Free, Illness-Free Series* to share accessible natural strategies that fit seamlessly into busy lives. His approach blends ancient healing principles with modern insight, helping people feel more energized, focused, and in tune with their long-term health goals.

Continue Your Wellness Journey

This book is just the beginning. True wellness is a lifelong journey, and you don't have to walk it alone. The Ashi Healing ecosystem is here to support you every step of the way with personalized guidance, nature-based solutions, and a shared mission: to help more people experience the benefits of natural health.

Personalized Virtual Consultation

If you're ready for expert guidance tailored to your specific needs, you can schedule a private virtual consultation with Dr. Forest Yin at AshiHealing.com. These one-on-one sessions offer a personalized supplement and herbal plan based on your current wellness goals, lifestyle, and health history, helping you create a sustainable path forward using time-tested, natural approaches.

In-Person Consultation and Acupuncture

If you're located in the San Francisco Bay Area, Dr. Yin also provides in-person consultations and acupuncture sessions at the University of East West Medicine (UEWM) campus in Sunnyvale, California, where he also teaches in the doctoral program for Traditional Chinese Medicine. This serene, professional setting offers a welcoming space for personalized care. All visits, virtual or in-person, can be scheduled through AshiHealing.com.

Supplement Recommendation Plans

Each wellness protocol discussed in this book has a corresponding supplement plan available on Fullscript, featuring practitioner-trusted, food-based formulas. These curated plans make it easy to take action without guesswork, offering clear, guided steps for nutritional support.

You can access them directly at:

https://us.fullscript.com/welcome/ashi-healing,

or simply start from AshiHealing.com.

Explore the Complete Book Series

This book is part of *The Medicine-Free, Illness-Free Series*, a 10-book collection designed to help you support your long-term health and vitality through natural methods. Each volume introduces a unique modality—from herbs and mushrooms to detoxification, grounding, amino acids, and more—so you can build your wellness path one step at a time.

Refer to the Series Overview chapter or visit AshiHealing.com to explore the full collection.

Support the Natural Health Movement

If this book has inspired you, and you believe more people should have access to clear, trustworthy information about natural health, consider supporting our mission.

The Ashi Healing Foundation *(AshiHealing.org)* is a nonprofit organization dedicated to public education, natural health awareness, and holistic wellness outreach. Your tax-deductible donation helps expand access to these tools and empowers more individuals to explore safe, evidence-informed approaches to well-being.

To contribute, visit AshiHealing.org and join the movement for a healthier, freer world.

Connect and Stay Inspired

Your healing journey doesn't end here.

Follow **Dr. Forest Yin** for more healing stories, tips, and inspiration:

Instagram, TikTok, YouTube, and X: @DrForestYin

Facebook: @DrForestYin1

LinkedIn: linkedin.com/in/forest-yin

Ready to Take the Next Step?

Scan the QR code below to visit AshiHealing.com, your starting point for virtual consultations, supplement plans, and more resources.

Your journey toward sustainable, natural wellness begins now.

'